Official Journal of the International Society of Nutrigenetics/Nutrigenomics (ISNN)

Journal of Nutrigenetics and Nutrigenomics

KARGER

Printed in Switzerland on acid-free and non-aging paper (ISO 9706) by Reinhardt Druck, Basel

Appears bimonthly: 1 volume per year (6 issues)

Guidelines for Authors

Journal of
Nutrigenetics and Nutrigenomics

Aims and Scope

The emerging field of nutrigenetics and nutrigenomics is rapidly gaining importance, and this new international journal has been established to meet the needs of the investigators for a high-quality platform for their research. Endorsed by the recently founded 'International Society of Nutrigenetics and Nutrigenomics', the 'Journal of Nutrigenetics and Nutrigenomics' welcomes contributions not only investigating the role of genetic variation in response to diet and that of nutrients in the regulation of gene expression, but is also open for articles covering all aspects of gene-environment interactions in the determination of health and disease. Original papers and reviews cover the genetic basis for the variable responses to diet and lifestyle factors in chronic conditions (e.g. cardiovascular disease, obesity, diabetes, cancer), methods to assess gene-environment interactions and other related relevant topics, with research drawing from both human and animal studies.

Submission

Manuscripts written in English should be submitted online at:

www.karger.com/jnn

Should you experience problems with your submission, please contact:

Louis Pérusse, PhD
Associate Professor
Director, Division of Kinesiology
Dept. Preventive Medicine
Laval University – PEPS Bldg.
Ste-Foy, Quebec G1K 7P4
Canada
Tel. +1 (418) 656-7831
Fax +1 (418) 656-3044
E-Mail Louis.Perusse@kin.msp.ulaval.ca

Conditions

All manuscripts are subject to editorial review. Manuscripts are received with the explicit understanding that they are not under simultaneous consideration by any other publication. Submission of an article for publication implies transfer of the copyright from the author to the publisher upon acceptance. Accepted papers become the permanent property of 'Journal of Nutrigenetics and Nutrigenomics' and may not be reproduced by any means, in whole or in part, without the written consent of the publisher. It is the author's responsibility to obtain permission to reproduce illustrations, tables, etc. from other publications.

Authorship

Each author must have participated substantially in the work to take public responsibility for the content of the paper, and must give final approval of the final version of the manuscript.

Categories of Manuscripts

Original Papers are full-length research papers, from both human and animal studies, which cover topics relevant to gene-environment interactions: the genetic basis for variability in the response to diet and other indicators of lifestyle (e.g. exercise, smoking) in chronic diseases such as cardiovascular disease, obesity, diabetes, and cancer; the regulation of gene expression by nutrients; methods to assess gene-environment interactions. Other topics related to the above could be considered by contacting the Editor.

Review Papers are state-of-the art reviews in areas relevant to the field of nutrigenetics and nutrigenomics. Reviews may be invited by the Editor or may be submitted for consideration.

Editorials provide comments on papers published in 'Journal of Nutrigenetics and Nutrigenomics'. Editorials are usually invited by the Editors.

Special Requirements

1. Investigations Involving Human Subjects: 'Journal of Nutrigenetics and Nutrigenomics' requires that investigations performed on human subjects have the prior approval of the institutional committee on human experimentation. Authors are required to submit a signed statement as to the date and details of the appropriate review. In countries where such mechanisms for approval do not exist, authors are required to submit a signed declaration that the research was carried out in accordance with the Helsinki Declaration. A similar assurance is required to document that animal experimentation was performed under appropriate circumstances.

2. Statement for Authors Submitting Original Research or Case Reports: 'The enclosed manuscript ... (Title) ... has been approved by me as well as by the responsible authorities at the institute where the work has been carried out. I certify that none of the material in this manuscript has been published previously in any form and that none of this material is currently under consideration for publication elsewhere. This includes symposia and proceedings of meetings and preliminary publications of any kind except an abstract of 400 words or less.' (To be signed by *all* authors.)

3. The undersigned also confirm that they qualify for (co-) authorship according to the 'Uniform Requirements for Manuscripts' published in the guidelines of the 'International Committee of Medical Journal Editors' in 1988 as follows: Authorship credit should be based only on substantial contributions to (a) conception and design, or analysis and interpretation of data; (b) drafting the article or revising it critically for important intellectual content; and on (c) final approval of the version to be published. Conditions (a), (b), and (c) must all be met. Participation solely in the acquisition of funding or the collection of data does not justify authorship. General supervision of the research group is also not sufficient for authorship. Any part of an article critical to its main conclusions must be the responsibility of at least one author. Persons who have contributed intellectually to the article but whose contributions do not justify authorship may be named and their particular contribution described in the section 'Acknowledgements'. Such persons must give their permission to be named.

Arrangement

Title page: The first page of each paper should indicate the title, the authors' names, the institute where the work was conducted, and a short title for use as running head.
NB: Authors wishing to preserve the phonetic meaning of diacritics (PubMed reduces diacritics to their root characters) must spell their names accordingly when submitting manuscripts (e.g. Müller should be Mueller).

Full address: The exact postal address of the corresponding author complete with postal code must be given at the bottom of the title page. Please also supply phone and fax numbers, as well as e-mail address.

Key words: For indexing purposes, a list of 3–10 key words in English is essential.

Abstract: Each paper needs an abstract of up to 200 words. It should be structured as follows:

Background/Aims:	What is the major problem that prompted the study?
Methods:	How was the study performed?
Results:	Most important findings?
Conclusion:	Most important conclusion?

Footnotes: Avoid footnotes.

Tables and illustrations: Tables and illustrations (both numbered in Arabic numerals) should be prepared on separate pages. Tables require a heading and figures a legend, also prepared on a separate page. Due to technical reasons, figures with a screen background should not be submitted. When possible, group several illustrations in one block for reproduction (max. size 180 × 223 mm) or provide crop marks. Each illustration must be labelled with its number and the first author's name. B/w half-tone and color illustrations must have a final resolution of 300 dpi after scaling, line drawings one of 800–1,200 dpi. Figure files must not be embedded in a document file but submitted separately (see detailed instructions on the Submission Website at **www.karger.com/jnn**).

Color illustrations
Online edition: Color illustrations are reproduced free of charge. In the print version, the illustrations are reproduced in black and white. Please avoid referring to the colors in the text and figure legends.
Print edition: Up to 6 color illustrations per page can be integrated within the text at CHF 760.– per page.

References: In the text identify references by Arabic numerals [in square brackets]. Material submitted for publication but not yet accepted should be noted as 'unpublished data' and not be included in the reference list. The list of references should include only those publications which are cited in the text. Do not alphabetize; number references in the order in which they are first mentioned in the text. The surnames of the authors followed by initials should be given. There should be no punctuation other than a comma to separate the authors. Preferably, please cite all authors. Abbreviate journal names according to the Index Medicus system. (Also see International Committee of Medical Journal Editors: Uniform requirements for manuscripts submitted to biomedical journals. N Engl J Med 1997;336:309–315. www.icmje.org)

Digital Object Identifier (DOI)
S. Karger Publishers supports DOIs as unique identifiers for articles. A DOI number will be printed on the title page of each article. DOIs can be useful in the future for identifying and citing articles published online without volume or issue information. More information can be found at www.doi.org.

Examples
(a) Papers published in periodicals: Chatel J-M, Bernard H, Orson FM: Isolation and characterization of two complete Ara h 2 isoforms cDNA. Int Arch Allergy Immunol 2003;131:14–18.
(b) Papers published only with DOI numbers:
Theoharides TC, Boucher W, Spear K: Serum interleukin-6 reflects disease severity and osteoporosis in mastocytosis patients. Int Arch Allergy Immunol DOI: 10.1159/000063858.
(c) Monographs: Matthews DE, Farewell VT: Using and Understanding Medical Statistics, ed 3, revised. Basel, Karger, 1996.
(d) Edited books: DuBois RN: Cyclooxygenase-2 and colorectal cancer; in Dannenberg AJ, Dubois RN (eds): COX-2. Prog Exp Tum Res. Basel, Karger, 2003, vol 37, pp 124–137.

Author's Choice™

With this option the author can choose to make his article freely available online against a one-time fee of CHF 2750.–. This fee is independent of any standard charges for supplementary pages, color images etc. which may apply. More information can be found at www.karger.com/authors_choice.

Page Charges

There are no page charges for papers of 8 or fewer printed pages (including tables, illustrations and references). Each additional complete or partial page is charged to the author at CHF 290.–. The allotted size of a paper is equal to approx. 20 manuscript pages (including tables, illustrations and references). The inability to pay the additional page charges will not prejudice publication of the paper. This will be decided by the Editor.

Proofs

Unless indicated otherwise, proofs are sent to the first-named author and should be returned with the least possible delay. Alterations made in proofs, other than the correction of printer's errors, are charged to the author.

Reprints

Order forms and a price list are sent with the proofs. Orders submitted after the issue is printed are subject to considerably higher prices.

KARGER
Fax +41 61 306 12 34
E-Mail karger@karger.ch
www.karger.com

The Guidelines for Authors are available at:
www.karger.com/jnn_Guidelines

General Information

ISSN Print Edition: 1661–6499
ISSN Online Edition: 1661–6758

Journal Homepage: www.karger.com/jnn

Publication Data: 'Journal of Nutrigenetics and Nutrigenomics' is published 6 times a year. Volume 1 with 6 issues appears in 2008.

Disclaimer: The statements, options and data contained in this publication are solely those of the individual authors and contributors and not of the publisher and the editor(s). The appearance of advertisements in the journal is not a warranty, endorsement, or approval of the products or services advertised or of their effectiveness, quality or safety. The publisher and the editor(s) disclaim responsibility for any injury to persons or property resulting from any ideas, methods, instructions or products referred to in the content or advertisements.

Subscription Rates: Subscriptions run for a full calendar year. Prices are given per year.

Personal subscription:

Print or Online	**Print+Online combined**
CHF 394.80	CHF 439.80
EUR 282.–	EUR 314.–
USD 358.80	USD 399.80

postage and handling (added to print and print+online)
CHF 36.– Europe, CHF 54.– Overseas
EUR 25.80
USD 49.50

Institutional subscription:

Print or Online	**Print+Online combined**
CHF 987.–	CHF 1086.–
EUR 705.–	EUR 776.–
USD 897.00	USD 987.00

postage and handling (added to print and print+online)
CHF 45.– Europe, CHF 67.50 Overseas
EUR 32.40
USD 61.80

Airmail surcharge: CHF 45.60 / USD 41.40

Discount subscription prices:
The 'Journal of Nutrigenetics and Nutrigenomics' is included in the 'International Society of Nutrigenetics/Nutrigenomics (ISNN)' membership fee, for information: **www.issn.info**

Back Volumes and Single Issues: Information on availability and prices of single print issues and print or electronic back volumes can be obtained from Customer Service at *service@karger.ch.*

Photocopying: This journal has been registered with the Copyright Clearance Center (CCC), as indicated by the code appearing on the first page of each article. For readers in the US, this code signals consent for copying of articles for personal or internal use, or for the personal or internal use of specific clients, provided that the stated fee is paid per copy directly to
Copyright Clearance Center Inc.
222 Rosewood Drive
Danvers, MA 01923 (USA)
A copy of the first page of the article must accompany payment. Consent does not extend to copying for general distribution, for promotion, for creating new works, or for resale. In these cases, specific written permission must be obtained from the copyright owner,
S. Karger AG, P.O. Box
CH–4009 Basel (Switzerland).

Subscription Orders:
Orders can be placed at agencies, bookstores, directly with the Publisher

S. Karger AG
Medical and Scientific Publishers
P.O. Box
CH–4009 Basel
Switzerland
(for courier services only:
Allschwilerstrasse 10
CH–4055 Basel)
Tel. +41 61 306 11 11
Fax +41 61 306 12 34
E-Mail karger@karger.ch
www.karger.com

or further Karger offices or representatives:

France:
Librairie Medi-Sciences Sarl
36, bd de Latour-Maubourg
75007 Paris
France
Tél. +33 (0) 1 45 51 42 58
Fax +33 (0) 1 45 56 07 80
E-Mail librairie@medi-sciences.fr
www.medi-sciences.fr

Germany:
S. Karger GmbH
Postfach
79095 Freiburg
Deutschland
(Hausadresse: Lörracher Strasse 16A
79115 Freiburg)
Tel. +49 761 45 20 70
Fax +49 761 45 20 714
E-Post information@karger.de
www.karger.de

India, Bangladesh, Sri Lanka:
Panther Publishers Private Ltd.
33, First Main
Koramangala First Block
Bangalore 560 034
India
Tel. +91 80 25505 836
Tel. +91 80 25505 837
Fax +91 80 25505 981
E-Mail panther_publishers@vsnl.com
www.pantherpublishers.com

Japan:
Karger Japan, Inc.
Yushima S Bld. 3F
4-2-3, Yushima, Bunkyo-ku
Tokyo 113-0034
Japan
Tel. +81 3 3815 1800
Fax +81 3 3815 1802
E-Mail publisher@karger.jp

China, Taiwan and Malaysia:
Karger China
Mr. Raymond Chew
Suite 409, Apollo Building
1440 Central Yan An Road
Shanghai 200040
China
Tel. +86-21-6133 1861
Fax +86-21-6133 1862
E-Mail karger.ray@gmail.com

South America and Central America:
Cranbury International LLC
7 Clarendon Ave., Suite 2
Montpelier, VT 05602
USA
Tel. +1 802 223 6565
Fax +1 802 223 6824
E-Mail
eatkin@cranburyinternational.com
www.cranburyinternational.com

United Kingdom, Ireland:
S. Karger AG
c/o London Liaison Office
4 Rickett Street
London SW6 1RU
United Kingdom
Tel. +44 (0) 20 7386 0500
Fax +44 (0) 20 7610 3337
E-Mail uk@karger.ch

USA:
S. Karger Publishers, Inc.
26 West Avon Road
P.O. Box 529
Unionville, CT 06085
USA
Toll free: +1 800 828 5479
Tel. +1 860 675-7834
Fax +1 860 675-7302
E-Mail karger@snet.net

Change of Address:
Both old and new address should be sent to the subscription source.

KARGER

Fax +41 61 306 12 34
E-Mail karger@karger.ch
www.karger.com

The Journal Home Page is available at:
www.karger.com/jnn

Journal of
Nutrigenetics
and
Nutrigenomics

Genetic and Nutritional Determinants of the Metabolic Syndrome

Guest Editor
Jean-Pierre Després, Québec, Qué.

1 figure and 3 tables, 2008

KARGER

Basel · Freiburg · Paris · London · New York · Bangalore · Bangkok · Shanghai · Singapore · Tokyo · Sydney

S. Karger
Medical and Scientific Publishers
Basel • Freiburg • Paris • London
New York • Bangalore • Bangkok
Shanghai • Singapore • Tokyo • Sydney

Printed in Switzerland
on acid-free and non-aging paper (ISO 9706) by
Reinhardt Druck, Basel
ISBN 978–3–8055–8453–1

KARGER

Fax +41 61 306 12 34
E-Mail karger@karger.ch
www.karger.com

Vol. 1, No. 3, 2008

Journal of
Nutrigenetics
and
Nutrigenomics

Contents

KARGER

Fax +41 61 306 12 34
E-Mail karger@karger.ch
www.karger.com

Access to full text and tables of contents, including tentative ones for forthcoming issues: www.karger.com/jnn_issues

Journal of
Nutrigenetics and Nutrigenomics

J Nutrigenet Nutrigenomics 2008;1:97–99
DOI: 10.1159/000112456

Published online: February 20, 2008

Genetic and Nutritional Determinants of the Metabolic Syndrome: Introduction

Jean-Pierre Després[a, b] Louis Pérusse[b]

[a]Hôpital Laval Research Centre, and [b]Division of Kinesiology, Department of Social and Preventive Medicine, Université Laval, Québec, Qué., Canada

This issue of the *Journal of Nutrigenetics and Nutrigenomics* is devoted to an important public health and clinical issue: the metabolic syndrome. Although the metabolic syndrome has been defined as a cluster of metabolic abnormalities that is predictive of an increased risk of type-2 diabetes and cardiovascular disease, considerable confusion and debate remain around its definition and on the proper approach to diagnose the metabolic syndrome in clinical practice. In this regard, it is important to make the distinction between the definition of the metabolic syndrome as conceptualized by the National Cholesterol Education Program-Adult Treatment Panel III (NCEP-ATP III) guidelines versus the clinical tools that have been proposed to help health professionals diagnose this condition [1]. In this regard, it should be kept in mind that the metabolic syndrome has been defined by a cluster of athero-thrombotic-inflammatory abnormalities for which insulin resistance is a central key disturbance [2]. Furthermore, the NCEP-ATP III has proposed that abdominal obesity is the most prevalent form of insulin resistance in clinical practice [2]. Thus, the most prevalent form of the metabolic syndrome and insulin resistance is found in patients with abdominal obesity, insulin resistance and with an excess of visceral/ectopic fat [3]. If we consider this cluster as a prevalent form of insulin resistance, the metabolic syndrome may therefore represent a good disease model for nutrigenetic and nutrigenomic studies because there is now considerable evidence showing that (1) genetic variation influences the relationships between diets and the various clinical features of the metabolic syndrome, and (2) nutrients, especially dietary fat, could influence the expression of several genes associated with the various metabolic components of the metabolic syndrome through their binding with a class of nuclear receptors called peroxisome proliferator-activated receptors (PPARs). This special issue presents five papers that address the contributions of genetic and nutritional factors in the etiology of the metabolic syndrome as well as their interactions.

The first paper by Lévesque and Lamarche presents an overview of the various criteria that have been proposed by different organizations to diagnose the metabolic syndrome and provides data on the prevalence of the syndrome based on the various approaches and criteria. Despite slight differences between the proposed approaches, the majority of them reflect most of the clinical features encountered in the metabolic syndrome, which include insulin resistance or hyperglycemia, obesity or abdominal obesity, hypertension and dyslipidemia. The clinical relevance of the metabolic syndrome is discussed in the context of its usefulness to predict cardiovascular disease risk. Finally, the management of its various underlying risk factors is discussed.

In the second paper, Josse et al. present an overview of the various types of diets, nutrients and food components which have been shown to improve the various determinants of the metabolic syndrome. The role of very low calorie diets (VLCDs), high fat diets, low carbohydrate

KARGER

Fax +41 61 306 12 34
E-Mail karger@karger.ch
www.karger.com

1661–6499/08/0013–0097$24.50/0

Accessible online at:
www.karger.com/jnn

Jean-Pierre Després, PhD, FAHA
Québec Heart Institute, Hôpital Laval Research Centre, Hôpital Laval
2725, chemin Ste-Foy, Pavilion Marguerite-D'Youville, 4th Floor
Québec, Qué. G1V 4G5 (Canada)
Tel. +1 418 656 4863, Fax +1 418 656 4610, E-Mail jean-pierre.despres@crhl.ulaval.ca

diets, carbohydrates, fiber and whole grains, soy and nuts and glycemic index on insulin sensitivity and other features of the metabolic syndrome are reviewed.

The third paper by Lahiry et al. provides an overview of the genes predisposing to or protecting from the development of the metabolic syndrome. The paper reviews the results of candidate gene studies, genome-wide linkage and association studies. Genes associated with familial partial lipodystrophy, a monogenic disorder which is a relevant model for the study of a phenotype sharing some striking similarities with the clinical manifestations of the metabolic syndrome are also reviewed.

The fourth paper by Guri et al., presents a comprehensive review of the role of the PPARs and their role, as endogenous receptors of fatty acids and lipid metabolites, in the metabolic and inflammatory processes associated with the metabolic syndrome. The roles of PPARs in adipocyte hypertrophy, regulation of glucose utilization, macrophage infiltration into adipose tissue and macrophage function and lipoprotein metabolism are reviewed.

Finally, the last paper by Phillips et al., addresses the issue of gene–nutrient interactions in the metabolic syndrome. The authors present a brief review of the genetic determinants of the metabolic syndrome with an emphasis on the recent genome-wide association studies which have led to the identification of several important susceptibility genes for type-2 diabetes mellitus. The evidence of gene–nutrient interactions (with particular emphasis on dietary fatty acids) for the various components of the syndrome is then reviewed.

From the topics addressed in this issue, it is clear that the metabolic syndrome, whichever the criteria used to make its diagnosis, is predictive of an increased risk of type-2 diabetes and cardiovascular disease [4, 5]. However, the metabolic syndrome is not sufficient in itself to properly assess global risk of cardiovascular disease and attention should also be given to the presence of classical risk factors using global risk assessment algorithms such as the Framingham risk score. The overall cardiovascular risk resulting from the presence of the metabolic syndrome and classical risk factors has been defined as global cardiometabolic risk [3]. New, improved global risk assessment algorithms should be developed to capture the additional burden of the metabolic syndrome.

Clearly, one major positive implication around the proposal to assess the metabolic syndrome was to be able to emphasize to patients the importance of weight loss through improved nutrition and increased physical activity/exercise. The paper by Josse et al. provides evidence that the metabolic profile of patients could be substantially improved if we could reshape the nutritional habits of patients with the metabolic syndrome. Unfortunately, until we systematically include dieticians and kinesiologists and offer regular access to such teams of health professionals to our patients, there is little chance that we will be successful in having a significant impact on the cardiometabolic risk profile of sedentary, abdominally obese patients with the metabolic syndrome.

In the study of genetic factors involved in its development, the fact that various combinations of clinical criteria (3 of 5) can be used to diagnose the metabolic syndrome makes the study of its pathophysiology a rather daunting task. For instance, the abdominally obese, diabetic, hypertensive patient without high triglyceride-low HDL cholesterol dyslipidemia is likely to be metabolically distinct from the nondiabetic, normotensive abdominally obese patient with the atherogenic dyslipidemia of the metabolic syndrome. However, under our current clinical approaches, they would be considered as having the metabolic syndrome. Thus, some metabolic patients may be more prone to hypertension, others to diabetes, others to dyslipidemia whereas some patients may have the full-blown profile and have all the above complications. Clearly, the underlying metabolic defects may differ and a better characterization of metabolic syndrome sub-phenotypes will allow investigators to identify clear signals. Thus, the proper phenotyping of metabolic syndrome patients represents a challenge to the field.

However, there is substantial evidence suggesting that dysfunctional subcutaneous adipose tissue may be an important underlying abnormality leading to 'lipid overflow' and to ectopic fat deposition [3]. Under this model, a partially lipodystrophic patient without a proper 'metabolic sink' to clear the excess energy from the diet could not store this energy in subcutaneous adipose tissue, leading to the development of insulin resistance and the metabolic syndrome. As PPAR-γ receptors play a key role in the proliferation of adipose tissue, they certainly represent a very important target for genetic and metabolic studies.

Finally, although it is clear that some prevalent forms of the metabolic syndrome have a genetic component, how these various subgroups of patients with the metabolic syndrome respond to standardized environment changes is a key area with huge therapeutic implications. If we eventually wish to provide clear recommendations to the public and patients, we need to better characterize subgroups of susceptible individuals. Clearly, there will be low responders and high responders to lifestyle changes and we need to understand the mechanisms responsible for such heterogeneity of response, in order to develop individual approaches tailored to the patient's genotype/phenotype.

Thus, although its clinical diagnosis remains a challenge, the introduction of the metabolic syndrome concept has been a huge advance as we now recognize that there are sedentary, abdominally obese individuals who may develop various combinations of a constellation of metabolic abnormalities causing prejudice to their metabolic and cardiovascular health. The present issue discusses several important notions relevant to the pathophysiology and management of this prevalent condition. Clearly, more should be done to better understand the genetic factors involved in the etiology of common and less common forms of the metabolic syndrome, with proper consideration given to management approaches adjusted to the patient's genotype/phenotype.

Disclosure Statement

J.-P.D. received honoraria from: Abbott Laboratories; AstraZeneca; Fournier Pharma Inc./Solvay Pharma; GlaxoSmithKline; MSD; Pfizer Canada Inc.; Sanofi-Aventis; Novartis, and Innodia, as a consultant or lecturer. Furthermore, his laboratory received research grants from some of the aforementioned companies and also from the *Canadian Diabetes Association* and the *Canadian Institutes of Health Research.*

References

1 Després JP: Is visceral obesity the cause of the metabolic syndrome? Ann Med 2006;38:52–63.
2 Grundy SM, Cleeman JI, Daniels SR, Donato KA, Eckel RH, Franklin BA, Gordon DJ, Krauss RM, Savage PJ, Smith SC Jr, Spertus JA, Costa F: Diagnosis and management of the metabolic syndrome: an American Heart Association/National Heart, Lung, and Blood Institute Scientific Statement. Circulation 2005;112:2735–2752.
3 Després JP, Lemieux I: Abdominal obesity and metabolic syndrome. Nature 2006;444:881–887.
4 Galassi A, Reynolds K, He J: Metabolic syndrome and risk of cardiovascular disease: a meta-analysis. Am J Med 2006;119:812–819.
5 Gami AS, Witt BJ, Howard DE, Erwin PJ, Gami LA, Somers VK, Montori VM: Metabolic syndrome and risk of incident cardiovascular events and death: a systematic review and meta-analysis of longitudinal studies. J Am Coll Cardiol 2007;49:403–414.

Journal of
Nutrigenetics
and
Nutrigenomics

J Nutrigenet Nutrigenomics 2008;1:100–108
DOI: 10.1159/000112457

Published online: February 20, 2008

The Metabolic Syndrome: Definitions, Prevalence and Management

Josée Levesque Benoît Lamarche

Institute on Nutraceuticals and Functional Foods, Laval University, Québec, Qué., Canada

Key Words

Metabolic syndrome, definition · Insulin resistance syndrome · Obesity, prevalence and management

Abstract

The metabolic syndrome (MetS) refers to the clustering of various metabolic risk factors that include abdominal obesity, dyslipidemia, hypertension, and hyperglycemia. It is now well known that it is associated with an increased risk of cardiovascular disease (CVD) and of type 2 diabetes. The increasing prevalence of the MetS, associated with the substantial progression of obesity and diabetes, is therefore an important public health concern. Over the years, several definitions for the MetS have been proposed by major scientific associations. Those definitions differ somewhat in their criteria and threshold values but generally all agree on the essential components of the syndrome. The proposed definitions are intended to help identify individuals at increased long-term risk of CVD, who could benefit from early prevention. The diagnosis of the MetS should be used concurrently with standard predicting algorithms, such as the Framingham Risk Score and the Diabetes Predicting Model, which better predict short-term risks. The management of the MetS should emphasize therapeutic lifestyle modifications – weight loss, increased physical activity, healthy diet – as the first-line therapy. If the short-term risk of CVD or diabetes is high, specific risk factors should be monitored more closely according to established guidelines and drug therapy may be appropriate.

Introduction

The metabolic syndrome (MetS) is a cluster of metabolic abnormalities that predispose an individual to a greater risk of developing type 2 diabetes [1] and cardiovascular disease (CVD) [2, 3]. The concept of MetS, also known as the insulin resistance syndrome [4], syndrome X [5], and the deadly quartet [6], may have been introduced as early as 1923 by Kylin [7] as the clustering of hypertension, hyperglycemia, and hyperuricemia. The MetS was more comprehensively described in 1988 by Reaven [5] as a syndrome implying a dysregulated glucose and insulin homeostasis, but also comprising hypertension and a typical dyslipidemia characterized by elevated plasma triglyceride (TG) levels and low high-density lipoprotein cholesterol (HDL-C) concentrations. Abdominal obesity has since then been integrated by others as one of the key components of the MetS [8].

To help define the MetS for clinical and research purposes, diagnostic criteria have been proposed by different health organizations. Although the actual definitions differ somewhat in their criteria and threshold values, most agree on the essential components – obesity, dyslipidemia, hypertension, and glucose intolerance. Because of the notable interethnic differences in the obesity-associated risk of disease, several cutoff points have been proposed to adapt the definition of the MetS to different populations. Furthermore, the various available definitions share the same goal, to help identify high-risk individuals who would benefit from early and more intensive disease prevention.

KARGER

Fax +41 61 306 12 34
E-Mail karger@karger.ch
www.karger.com

1661–6499/08/0013–0100$24.50/0

Accessible online at:
www.karger.com/jnn

Benoît Lamarche, PhD
Institute on Nutraceuticals and Functional Foods
Pavillon des services, Laval University, 2440, Hochelaga Blvd
Québec, Qué, G1K 7P4 (Canada)
Tel. +1 418 656 3527, Fax +1 418 656 5877, E-Mail Benoit.Lamarche@inaf.ulaval.ca

Using different definitions, several studies have demonstrated that individuals with the MetS have a cardiovascular risk 2–5 times greater than those without the syndrome [2, 3, 9, 10]. The increasing worldwide prevalence of the MetS, an important public health concern, is intimately linked to the drastic progression of obesity and diabetes [11], and there is a sense of urgency within the medical and scientific community to develop strategies to slow down this emerging epidemic. It is yet not clear, however, which definition of the MetS best predicts the risk of future cardiovascular events.

The aim of this article is to provide an overview of the various definitions of the MetS, with emphasis on its increasing prevalence and its management.

Definitions of the Metabolic Syndrome

World Health Organization (1999)

The World Health Organization (WHO) Diabetes Group made the first attempt to define the MetS [12]. Diagnosis of the MetS based on this definition was primarily centered on the presence of insulin resistance as revealed by clamp studies, by diagnosis of impaired glucose tolerance or by relatively elevated plasma insulin levels, or type 2 diabetes. At least 2 of the following risk factors also needed to be present for a positive diagnosis: obesity (waist-to-hip ratio >0.90 for men and >0.85 for women and/or body mass index, BMI, >30), dyslipidemia (plasma TG concentrations ≥1.7 mmol/l and/or HDL-C levels <0.9 mmol/l for men and <1.0 mmol/l for women), hypertension (≥140/90 mm Hg), and microalbuminuria (urinary albumin excretion rate ≥20 μg/min or albumin:creatinine ratio ≥30 mg/g) [12].

European Group for the Study of Insulin Resistance (1999)

The same year, the European Group for the Study of Insulin Resistance (EGIR) recommended minor modifications to the WHO definition of the MetS in an attempt to make it simpler and easier to use. EGIR also suggested that the terminology 'insulin resistance syndrome' should be used. As in the WHO definition, insulin resistance, measured by clamp or estimated using fasting hyperinsulinemia defined as the upper quartile of a non-diabetic reference population, was a requirement for the diagnosis of the syndrome according to EGIR. However, because insulin resistance is such a strong risk factor for type 2 diabetes, they chose to exclude the diagnosis of type 2 diabetes as a criterion in their definition. In addition to insulin resistance, at least 2 of the following risk factors needed to be present: fasting hyperglycemia (≥6.1 mmol/l but below the diagnostic criteria for frank diabetes), hypertension (≥140/90 mm Hg) or treatment for hypertension, dyslipidemia (plasma TG concentrations ≥2.0 mmol/l and/or HDL-C levels <1.0 mmol/l) or treatment for dyslipidemia, and abdominal obesity (waist circumference ≥94 cm for men and ≥80 cm for women) [13]. The EGIR definition distinguished itself from the WHO definition by putting emphasis on central obesity rather than overall obesity, by discarding the criterion for microalbuminuria, and by including treatments for hypertension and dyslipidemia in the criteria of the corresponding abnormalities [13]. Cutoff points for most criteria were also different between the EGIR and WHO definitions of the MetS.

National Cholesterol Education Program – Adult Treatment Panel III (2001)

The third report of the National Cholesterol Education Program (NCEP) Expert Panel on Detection, Evaluation, and Treatment of High Blood Cholesterol in Adults (Adult Treatment Panel III; ATP III) proposed its own definition of the Mets in 2001. At least 3 of the following 5 risk factors needed to be present according to the NCEP-ATP III definition: abdominal obesity (waist circumference ≥102 cm for men and ≥88 cm for women), moderate hypertriglyceridemia (plasma TG concentrations ≥1.7 mmol/l), reduced HDL-C levels (<1.0 mmol/l for men and <1.3 mmol/l for women), hypertension (≥130/85 mm Hg), and fasting hyperglycemia (≥6.1 mmol/l) [8]. The cutoff points for the various criteria, excluding fasting glucose, are slightly different compared with previous definitions. In 2003, the American Diabetes Association lowered the cutoff point for impaired fasting glucose from 6.1 to 5.6 mmol/l [14] and the NCEP-ATP III definition of MetS was consequently modified [15]. Finally, as opposed to the WHO and EGIR definitions, the NCEP-ATP III definition of the MetS does not require the presence of insulin resistance.

American Association of Clinical Endocrinologists and the American College of Endocrinology (2003)

In 2003, the American Association of Clinical Endocrinologists (AACE) and the American College of Endocrinology (ACE) gave their definition for the MetS, which they also proposed should be referred to as the insulin resistance syndrome [16]. The blood pressure and lipid criteria of the NCEP-ATP III definition of the MetS were maintained. However, in addition to using fasting blood glucose, the use of an elevated 2-hour post-challenge glucose test was also encouraged. In contrast to previous definitions, AACE-ACE did not propose any criteria for obesity, which they suggested was a consequence of insulin resistance and/or hyperinsulinemia. The AACE-ACE definition also distinguished itself from the previous definitions by the absence of a numerical scoring of risk factors for the diagnosis of the insulin resistance syndrome, leaving the decision to the judgment of clinicians. This may be a major limitation to the widespread use of this definition. However, they proposed a series of risk factors that increase the probability of diagnosing the insulin resistance syndrome, including previously diagnosed CVD, non-Caucasian ethnicity, sedentary lifestyle, BMI >25 kg/m^2, age >40 years, polycystic ovary syndrome, and family history of type 2 diabetes, hypertension, or CVD [16].

International Diabetes Federation (2005)

In 2005, the International Diabetes Federation (IDF) made an attempt to unify the various definitions of the MetS [17]. The IDF definition does not require the presence of insulin resistance but emphasizes central obesity as assessed by the waist circumference. Indeed, an elevated waist girth is a mandatory criterion and the presence of at least 2 additional criteria confirms the diagnosis of the MetS. A unique feature of the IDF definition is the introduction of several ethnic-specific cutoff points for high waist circumference. The blood pressure and lipid criteria of the NCEP-ATP III definition of the MetS were maintained; treatments for dyslipidemia or hypertension and previously diagnosed type 2 diabetes were also considered diagnostic criteria. The impaired fasting glucose threshold was fixed at 5.6 mmol/l, in agreement with the new recommendations of the American Diabetes Association [14]. The IDF also recommended additional non-traditional criteria for research on the MetS, including biomarkers of adipose tissue (adiponectin, leptin), apolipoprotein B, low-density lipoprotein (LDL) particle size, endothelial dysfunction, urinary albumin, inflammatory markers (C-reactive protein (CRP), tumor necrosis factor, interleukin-6), and thrombotic markers (plasminogen activator inhibitor type 1, fibrinogen).

American Heart Association and the National Heart, Lung, and Blood Institute Statement on the Diagnosis and Management of the MetS (2005)

Shortly after the IDF proposed their new definition of the MetS, the American Heart Association (AHA) and the National Heart, Lung, and Blood Institute (NHLBI) issued a joint scientific statement on the diagnosis and management of the MetS [18]. Also based on the NCEP-ATP III definition, the AHA-NHLBI definition bears important similarities with the IDF definition. Hence, the criteria for hypertension, dyslipidemia, and impaired fasting glucose were comparable between the AHA-NHLBI and IDF definitions and treatments for corresponding abnormalities were also considered as diagnostic criteria. According to the AHA-NHLBI definition, and similar to the NCEP-ATP III definition, the diagnosis of the MetS requires the presence of at least 3 of the criteria and does not require the presence of any one particular criterion. Even though the AHA-NHLBI does not propose specific ethnic cutoff points for waist circumference, lower cutoff points are suggested for populations such as Asian Americans.

Hypertriglyceridemic Waist (2000)

Each feature of the MetS has been individually associated with an increased risk of CVD. Combination of specific non-traditional risk factors has also been proven to be strongly correlated with CVD risk beyond traditional risk factors. Specifically, the accumulation of these 3 non-traditional risk factors – namely small, dense, LDL particles, elevated plasma apolipoprotein (apo) B levels and elevated plasma insulin levels – has been associated with a >18-fold increase in the 5-year cardiovascular risk [19]. Because these non-traditional markers are not readily available to clinicians, our group developed the concept of the hypertriglyceridemic (hyperTG) waist, which strongly predicts the risk of carrying these 3 non-traditional risk factors. Thus, the hyperTG waist is defined by the presence of: (i) an elevated waist circumference ($\geq$90 cm in men), as a marker for elevated fasting insulin and apoB levels, and (ii) elevated plasma TG levels ($\geq$2.0 mmol/l), as a marker for small, dense, LDL particles [20]. Prospective large scale studies are needed to confirm the hyperTG waist phenotype's ability to predict future CVD events and type 2 diabetes onset.

Which Definition to Favor?

Over the years, the different definitions of the MetS have evolved, each definition bringing up novel perspectives on the syndrome while also intensifying the debate on which definition should be promoted in research as well as in clinical practice. The ideal definition of the MetS would be equally adequate and functional for clinical practice as well as for clinical, fundamental, and epidemiological research. It would also identify individuals at high risk of developing CVD as well as type 2 diabetes.

In clinical settings, a diagnostic tool must be simple to use, easily accessible and cost-effective. The hyperTG waist clearly appears as an ideal candidate, with only two components to integrate and manage. More prospective large scale studies are needed to establish this definition as a strong predictor of CVD and type 2 diabetes. As the next best choices, the NCEP-ATP III, the IDF, and the AHA-NHLBI definitions should be considered. These definitions appear to be simpler diagnostic definitions because they are based on criteria already being used in clinical practice. Therefore, these individual criteria can easily be regrouped in order to get a comprehensive overview on a patient's CVD and diabetes risks, as predicted by the MetS. The NCEP-ATP III definition has been extensively used compared to others and several large scale studies have confirmed its ability to predict both CVD and type 2 diabetes. However, these four definitions may be more specific to CVD than to type 2 diabetes because they do not formally require the presence of insulin resistance in their criteria, as do the WHO and the EGIR definitions. The AACE-ACE definition does not require the presence of insulin resistance but suggests that this is the underlying cause of the MetS [21].

In research settings, the definition of the MetS that will appear appropriate and optimal will depend on the objectives pursued by the research. In epidemiological research, simple and low-cost tools are needed to investigate large cohorts of subjects. Therefore, the same four definitions should be considered: the NCEP-ATP III, the IDF, and the AHA-NHLBI definitions, and the hyperTG waist. On the other hand, in clinical and smaller-scale human investigations, definitions could be extended and further detailed to include more specific components of the syndrome. The IDF definition is an interesting candidate because of the wide range in additional non-traditional criteria that were recommended for research on the MetS. Because the definition of the MetS is a work in progress, we believe that research should still not be restricted to any one specific definition [21].

Comparison of the Definitions of the Metabolic Syndrome

Comparison of the Estimated Prevalence of the Metabolic Syndrome

Independent of the different definitions and criteria used, it has been well demonstrated that the worldwide prevalence of the MetS is increasing, largely because of the rise in obesity rates. The prevalence of the MetS is also age-dependent. The National Health and Nutrition Examination Survey (NHANES) III was the first study to estimate the prevalence of the MetS among US adults. Using the NCEP-ATP III definition of the MetS, they found a prevalence of 6.7% among participants aged 20–29 years and of 43.5% among those aged 60–69 years [22]. Overall, the age-adjusted prevalence was similar for men (24.0%) and for women (23.4%) [22]. Ethnicity had a definite impact on the prevalence of MetS, the Mexican Americans having the highest age-adjusted prevalence (31.9%) and the African Americans and Caucasians the lowest prevalence (21.6 and 23.8%, respectively) [22]. It was also documented that metabolic abnormalities and the MetS are increasingly prevalent among US adolescents, a direct consequence of the increasing rates of obesity in younger age groups [23]. It is still debated which definition of the MetS, existing or modified, should be used in children and adolescents.

The comparison of the prevalence of the MetS in US adults using different definitions revealed that the overall prevalence was comparable using the WHO (25.1%) and the NCEP-ATP III definitions (23.9%) [24]. Although estimates using the WHO and NCEP-ATP III definitions were comparable among Caucasians, estimates differed more considerably for other ethnic groups. For example, the largest difference occurred among African American men, of whom 16.5% were classified as having the MetS using the NCEP-ATP III definition whereas 24.9% had the MetS using the WHO definition [24]. A study in Sweden revealed that the prevalence of MetS according to the IDF definition was slightly higher (21.9%) in comparison with the NCEP-ATP III (20.7%) and EGIR (18.8%) definitions [25]. In another European study, the prevalence of the MetS according to definitions from the WHO, the NCEP-ATP III, the NCEP-ATP III revised and the IDF was 27.0, 25.9, 32.2 and 35.9%, respectively, in men and 19.7, 23.4, 28.5 and 34.1%, respectively, in women [26]. Finally, the prevalence of the MetS using the IDF and AHA-NHLBI definitions in a population from Taiwan was relatively well correlated: 6.2 and 11.6%, respectively, in men, 12.6 and 16.5%, respectively, in women [27]. However, values were generally lower than those generated by previous studies using the WHO or the NCEP-ATP III definitions.

In summary, the IDF definition appears to predict a higher prevalence of the MetS compared with previously established definitions, when comparing prevalences within each study. On the other hand, the NCEP-ATP III definition appears to yield relatively consistent results in Caucasians, when comparing prevalences between different published studies.

Metabolic Syndrome Definitions and Cardiovascular Disease Risk Prediction

Several studies have attempted to evaluate which of the different MetS definitions would better predict the risk of CVD. A study in Sweden indicated that, even though the prevalence of MetS according to the IDF definition was higher than with NCEP-ATP III and EGIR definitions, the IDF definition was not superior in predicting the risk of CVD, a finding consistent within both genders [25]. Another European study compared estimates of CVD mortality rates derived from the WHO, NCEP-ATP III, NCEP-ATP III revised and IDF definitions. MetS, as diagnosed by these four definitions, predicted increased CVD mortality rates in men [26]. However, hazard ratios for men were higher with the WHO definition than with the IDF definition [26]. The hazard ratios for women were generally lower than those calculated for men, for every definition of the MetS used, except for the IDF definition, which yielded comparable hazard ratios in both genders [26]. These findings suggest gender differences in the MetS prediction of CVD mortality rates. The association between carotid atherosclerosis, a surrogate of CVD risk, and different MetS definitions (NCEP-ATP III, IDF and AHA-NHLBI) has also been evaluated. Regardless of the definition used, carotid intima-media thickness was significantly higher in both men and women diagnosed with the MetS compared to those without the MetS [28]. The strongest predictor of carotid atherosclerosis was the AHA-NHLBI definition in males, whereas it was the IDF definition in females [28]. Again, these results suggest important gender differences in the MetS definitions for the prediction of early atherosclerotic lesions [28]. In a Greek population, CVD prevalence was increased in the presence of MetS regardless of the definition used, but the increase was more pronounced with the NCEP-ATP III and AHA-NHLBI definitions compared with the IDF definition [29]. The IDF definition included a large proportion of subjects among whom CVD prevalence was comparable to the CVD prevalence among the entire study population [29]. In type 2 diabetic patients, the MetS prevalence was higher when using the IDF definition (73.7%) than with the NCEP-ATP III definition (68.4%) [30]. However, the diagnosis of MetS using the NCEP-ATP III definition was associated with higher all-cause mortality rates, while the association for the IDF definition was not significant [30]. It was therefore concluded that in a population at high risk with type 2 diabetes, the use of the IDF definition predicts a higher prevalence of the MetS, without improving its prognostic value on the risk of mortality [30].

In summary, only a few published studies have compared different MetS definitions as predictors of CVD development or mortality. According to most studies, the IDF definition of the MetS appears to be a less powerful predictor of CVD prognosis. Gender differences for the prediction of CVD risk with various definitions were also highlighted. Finally, it must be stressed that many of the previously described studies were conducted in European or Asian populations. Because of significant ethnic differences in the development of the MetS and its association with disease onset, the relevance and applicability of many of these studies to North American populations may be questioned.

Management of the Metabolic Syndrome

The clinical relevance of the MetS was challenged by a study that has compared the MetS definition and the Diabetes Predicting Model and the Framingham Risk Score as methods for identifying high-risk individuals for type 2 diabetes and CVD, respectively [31]. Data indicated that the MetS definition was inferior to these two established predicting models for the prediction of their related outcomes. This fuelled the debate on whether or not the cluster of MetS risk factors confers a higher cardiovascular risk than the sum of its individual components [32]. The joint AHA-NHLBI statement has re-emphasized the importance of considering the MetS as a clinical entity, based on the arguments that the Diabetes Predicting Model and the Framingham Risk Score are best at identifying short-term risk (<10 years), whereas MetS definitions would predict a longer-term risk of disease [18]. Therefore, the clinical usefulness of the MetS diagnosis may be in identifying, at an early stage, individuals at high long-term risk of CVD rather than short-term risk, as determined by traditional predicting models [33]. After assessment of the 10-year risk for CVD, if the short-term risk is low in a patient with the MetS, therapeutic lifestyle modifications are the first-line therapy to attenuate its associated long-term risk [8]. On the other hand, if the short-term risk is high, drug therapy is likely to be required to modify specific cardiovascular risk factors.

Management of Underling Risk Factors

The first step in the management of the MetS is to control underling modifiable risk factors, principally obesity, physical inactivity, and an atherogenic diet [34]. These therapeutic lifestyle modifications should be recommended to every person diagnosed with the MetS, independent of their risk assessment, because they are basically healthy lifestyle habits. Obesity, physical inactivity and poor diet are also most likely key etiological factors leading to the development of the MetS.

Overweight, Physical Inactivity/Sedentary Lifestyle and Dietary Modifications

Abdominal obesity is very closely associated with the MetS and many of its underlying risk factors [8]. Obesity guidelines [35] insist on weight reduction through behavioral changes to reduce caloric intake and increase physical activity, in order to achieve a 7–10% weight loss over 6–12 months. Because extreme diets are usually not effective in producing a long-term weight loss, the most effective weight loss strategy has been shown to be a modest 500- to 1,000-calorie/day reduction. Bariatric surgery conveys interesting results among morbidly obese patients with the MetS. A significant weight reduction 1 year after the surgery improved all the features of the MetS and resulted in a cure rate of 95.6% [36]. The daily physical exercise recommendation is 30 min of physical activity of moderate intensity [37]. Long-term maintenance of the weight loss is more successful by increasing regular physical exercise [35]. Finally, individuals with the MetS should also adhere to the following basic dietary principles: low intakes of saturated fats, *trans* fats, and cholesterol, reduced consumption of simple sugars, and increased intakes of fruits, vegetables, and whole grains [8]. The relative proportions of dietary carbohydrates and fat (low-fat/high-carbohydrates vs. low-carbohydrates/high-fat diets) for optimal long-term management of the MetS and its risk factors remains an issue of intense debate [34]. Therapeutic lifestyle modifications have been shown to prevent the development of type 2 diabetes in high-risk individuals. In subjects with impaired glucose tolerance, lifestyle changes have been proven to reduce the incidence of diabetes by 58% after 4 years [38]. In non-diabetic individuals with elevated fasting and post-load plasma glucose concentrations, lifestyle modifications and metformin both reduced the incidence of diabetes, but lifestyle changes were significantly more effective than metformin [39].

Management of Metabolic Risk Factors

Therapeutic lifestyle modifications improve the severity of most of the risk factors associated with the MetS [8] and therefore should precede the management of the individual metabolic risk factors. A pharmacological agent called rimonabant, a cannabinoid (CB_1) receptor blocker that is under investigation, has been shown to significantly reduce body weight (–6.7 ± 0.5 kg), reduce waist circumference (–5.8 ± 0.5 cm), and improve the metabolic risk profile in high-risk overweight or obese patients with atherogenic dyslipidemia, over one year as compared with placebo [40]. However, until its efficacy is further confirmed, treatment of the different risk factors through drug therapy should follow current guidelines for each individual risk factor.

Atherogenic Dyslipidemia

The MetS is associated with atherogenic dyslipidemia, which is characterized by elevated TG and apoB levels, small dense LDL particles, and low HDL-C concentrations [34]. Statins are widely used to reduce the risk of cardiovascular events. The cardiovascular benefits of statin therapy are mostly produced by their powerful cholesterol-lowering properties but also by pleiotropic effects independent of cholesterol reductions [41]. Fibrates more specifically target atherogenic dyslipidemia by significantly reducing plasma TG levels and moderately increasing HDL-C concentrations [8], but the efficacy of fibrates alone in reducing CVD events has not yet been substantiated, particularly among individuals with type 2 diabetes [42]. A subanalysis of the Veterans Affairs HDL Intervention Trial has shown that the group with insulin resistance at baseline experienced the greatest benefit from receiving a fibrate, gemfibrozil, in terms of a reduction in CVD rates [43]. The combined use of statin and fibrates produces the most beneficial effects on all lipid parameters and may result in the greatest improvement in CVD risk status [44]. Despite an increased risk of myopathy, such a combination remains an attractive avenue, especially if low doses are used [34].

Hypertension

Blood pressure reduction has important cardiovascular benefits, even in patients with type 2 diabetes [45, 46]. Blood pressure can be mildly reduced by several lifestyle changes, such as weight control, increased physical activity, alcohol moderation, sodium reduction, and increased consumption of fruits, vegetables and low-fat dairy products [18]. However, antihypertensive drugs are often required in addition to lifestyle changes to reach blood pressure goals [45]. Angiotensin-converting enzyme inhibitors or angiotensin receptor blockers are often the first-line therapy suggested, also in MetS and type 2 diabetic patients [47].

Insulin Resistance and Hyperglycemia

Metformin, thiazolidinediones and acarbose are used in the treatment of type 2 diabetes. Studies have investigated their efficacy to prevent diabetes in individuals with impaired glucose tolerance and impaired fasting glucose, and they have shown that theses drugs are effective at delaying type 2 diabetes onset [39, 48, 49]. Possibly because of the association between type 2 diabetes and CVD, it is suggested that these anti-diabetic drugs could also reduce and prevent CVD [49, 50]. It must be kept in mind that lipid-altering, antihypertensive, and hypoglycemic drugs sometimes have negative repercussions on body weight and insulin sensitivity [34]. Clinicians must therefore be careful in treating the MetS as a whole and aim for improvement in as many MetS features as possible.

Prothrombotic State

Although not included in the MetS criteria in most definitions, prothrombotic and pro-inflammatory states accompany the MetS most of the time and they will be briefly discussed. A prothrombotic state consists of an elevation in coagulation factors, such as fibrinogen and plasminogen activator inhibitor-1, and increases susceptibility to arterial thrombosis [34]. Low-dose aspirin or other anti-platelet drugs are recommended in secondary prevention of CVD [34], in primary prevention of CVD in type 2 diabetics [34], and in individuals with the MetS and a high risk of CVD [51].

Pro-Inflammatory State

A pro-inflammatory state is characterized by elevated cytokines (TNFα, IL-6) and acute phase reactants (CRP, fibrinogen) [34]. CRP is proposed to be a sensitive marker of subclinical inflammation, associated with the atherosclerosis process and CVD [52]. Studies have shown that individuals with elevated CRP concentrations (>3.0 mg/l) are more vulnerable to develop CVD than those with constitutive CRP concentrations below 1.0 mg/l [52]. Increased plasma CRP concentrations have been associated with many features of the MetS and, moreover, CRP concentrations increase as the number of components of the MetS also increases [53, 54]. This could result from the secretion by adipose tissue of several inflammatory cytokines, including IL-6, which stimulates CRP synthesis by the liver [55, 56]. Measurement of CRP among patients with the MetS has added significant prognostic information on cardiovascular risk at all levels of severity of the MetS [53], suggesting that addition of CRP to the current criteria used to diagnose the MetS should be considered. More research on this is still warranted. Although no specific anti-inflammatory drugs are available to treat a pro-inflammatory state, several drugs used to treat other metabolic risk factors have demonstrated anti-inflammatory properties. Indeed, statins, fibrates, and thiazolidinediones have been shown to reduce plasma CRP concentrations [57–60]. However, these drugs are not currently recommended solely to reduce a pro-inflammatory state independent of other risk factors [34].

Nutrigenomics and the Metabolic Syndrome

The physiopathology of the MetS remains unclear. The diversity of the MetS's metabolic abnormalities indicates that it is a multifactorial disease in which many genes may be implicated. Nutrigenomics, an emerging field of study where gene–nutrient interactions are investigated, represents an interesting avenue to gain new insight into the etiology of the MetS. The goal of nutrigenomics is to develop more specific population-based and even personalized dietary recommendations based on the genetic makeup of the individuals in order to prevent chronic diseases. The human genome has remained unchanged in the last decades but the prevalence of the MetS has drastically increased, indicating that important gene–environment interactions are at play [61]. Therapeutic lifestyle changes including healthy eating habits and weight loss significantly improve most metabolic abnormalities of the MetS. This confirms that nutrition as an environmental factor plays a key role in the development of the MetS. Finally, the MetS appears to have a component of heritability, which suggests a genetic basis [32]. This is evidenced by the wide interethnic differences in the development of abdominal obesity and the MetS. Thus, the association of population genomics with epidemiological population nutritional studies could help identify why certain populations are more susceptible to developing the MetS, CVD, and type 2 diabetes.

Conclusions

The rising prevalence of the MetS and its associated high risk of CVD and type 2 diabetes are major public health concerns. Because the Diabetes Predicting Model and the Framingham Risk Score have been shown to be superior to the MetS definition in identifying high-risk individuals for type 2 diabetes and CVD, respectively, the clinical relevance of using the MetS definitions has been questioned. However, these two established models are relatively accurate in predicting short-term risk (<10 years), whereas a diagnosis of MetS may predict a longer-term risk. Thus, the joint AHA-NHLBI statement has emphasized the important role of considering MetS in risk management. Challenges ahead include the development of a definition for the MetS that is sensitive enough to detect high-risk individuals earlier than can be achieved using existing prediction models.

Disclosure Statement

The authors declare that no financial or other conflict of interest exists in relation to the content of the article.

References

1 Grundy SM, Hansen B, Smith SC Jr, Cleeman JI, Kahn RA: Clinical management of metabolic syndrome: report of the American Heart Association/National Heart, Lung, and Blood Institute/American Diabetes Association conference on scientific issues related to management. Circulation 2004;109:551–556.

2 Lakka HM, Laaksonen DE, Lakka TA, Niskanen LK, Kumpusalo E, Tuomilehto J, Salonen JT: The metabolic syndrome and total and cardiovascular disease mortality in middle-aged men. JAMA 2002;288:2709–2716.

3 Isomaa B, Almgren P, Tuomi T, Forsen B, Lahti K, Nissen M, Taskinen MR, Groop L: Cardiovascular morbidity and mortality associated with the metabolic syndrome. Diabetes Care 2001;24:683–689.

4 DeFronzo RA, Ferrannini E: Insulin resistance. A multifaceted syndrome responsible for NIDDM, obesity, hypertension, dyslipidemia, and atherosclerotic cardiovascular disease. Diabetes Care 1991;14:173–194.

5 Reaven GM: Banting Lecture 1988. Role of insulin resistance in human disease. Diabetes 1988;37:1595–1607.

6 Kaplan NM: The deadly quartet. Upper-body obesity, glucose intolerance, hypertriglyceridemia, and hypertension. Arch Intern Med 1989;149:1514–1520.

7 Kylin E: Studien über das Hypertonie-Hyperglykämie-Hyperurikämiesyndrom. Zentralbl Inn Med 1923;44:105–127.

8 Executive Summary of the Third Report of the National Cholesterol Education Program (NCEP) Expert Panel on Detection, Evaluation, and Treatment of High Blood Cholesterol In Adults (Adult Treatment Panel III). JAMA 2001;285:2486–2497.

9 Howard BV, Criqui MH, Curb JD, Rodabough R, Safford MM, Santoro N, Wilson AC, Wylie-Rosett J: Risk factor clustering in the insulin resistance syndrome and its relationship to cardiovascular disease in postmenopausal white, black, hispanic, and Asian/Pacific Islander women. Metabolism 2003;52:362–371.

10 Resnick HE, Jones K, Ruotolo G, Jain AK, Henderson J, Lu W, Howard BV: Insulin resistance, the metabolic syndrome, and risk of incident cardiovascular disease in nondiabetic American Indians: the Strong Heart Study. Diabetes Care 2003;26:861–867.

11 Zimmet P, Alberti KG, Shaw J: Global and societal implications of the diabetes epidemic. Nature 2001;414:782–787.

12 WHO: Definition, Diagnosis and Classification of Diabetes Mellitus and Its Complications. Part I. Diagnosis and Classification of Diabetes Mellitus. Geneva, World Health Organization, 1999.

13 Balkau B, Charles MA: Comment on the provisional report from the WHO consultation. European Group for the Study of Insulin Resistance (EGIR). Diabet Med 1999;16:442–443.

14 Genuth S, Alberti KG, Bennett P, Buse J, Defronzo R, Kahn R, Kitzmiller J, Knowler WC, Lebovitz H, Lernmark A, Nathan D, Palmer J, Rizza R, Saudek C, Shaw J, Steffes M, Stern M, Tuomilehto J, Zimmet P: Follow-up report on the diagnosis of diabetes mellitus. Diabetes Care 2003;26:3160–3167.

15 Grundy SM, Brewer HB Jr, Cleeman JI, Smith SC Jr, Lenfant C: Definition of metabolic syndrome: report of the National Heart, Lung, and Blood Institute/American Heart Association conference on scientific issues related to definition. Circulation 2004;109:433–438.

16 Einhorn D, Reaven GM, Cobin RH, Ford E, Ganda OP, Handelsman Y, Hellman R, Jellinger PS, Kendall D, Krauss RM, Neufeld ND, Petak SM, Rodbard HW, Seibel JA, Smith DA, Wilson PW: American College of Endocrinology position statement on the insulin resistance syndrome. Endocr Pract 2003;9:237–252.

17 Alberti KG, Zimmet P, Shaw J: The metabolic syndrome – a new worldwide definition. Lancet 2005;366:1059–1062.

18 Grundy SM, Cleeman JI, Daniels SR, Donato KA, Eckel RH, Franklin BA, Gordon DJ, Krauss RM, Savage PJ, Smith SC Jr, Spertus JA, Costa F: Diagnosis and management of the metabolic syndrome: an American Heart Association/National Heart, Lung, and Blood Institute Scientific Statement. Circulation 2005;112:2735–2752.

19 Lamarche B, Tchernof A, Mauriege P, Cantin B, Dagenais GR, Lupien PJ, Despres JP: Fasting insulin and apolipoprotein B levels and low-density lipoprotein particle size as risk factors for ischemic heart disease. JAMA 1998;279:1955–1961.

20 Lemieux I, Pascot A, Couillard C, Lamarche B, Tchernof A, Almeras N, Bergeron J, Gaudet D, Tremblay G, Prud'homme D, Nadeau A, Despres JP: Hypertriglyceridemic waist: a marker of the atherogenic metabolic triad (hyperinsulinemia; hyperapolipoprotein B; small, dense LDL) in men? Circulation 2000;102:179–184.

21 Desroches S, Lamarche B: The evolving definitions and increasing prevalence of the metabolic syndrome. Appl Physiol Nutr Metab 2007;32:23–32.

22 Ford ES, Giles WH, Dietz WH: Prevalence of the metabolic syndrome among US adults: findings from the Third National Health and Nutrition Examination Survey. JAMA 2002;287:356–359.

23 de Ferranti SD, Gauvreau K, Ludwig DS, Newburger JW, Rifai N: Inflammation and changes in metabolic syndrome abnormalities in US adolescents: findings from the 1988–1994 and 1999–2000 National Health and Nutrition Examination Surveys. Clin Chem 2006;52:1325–1330.

24 Ford ES, Giles WH: A comparison of the prevalence of the metabolic syndrome using two proposed definitions. Diabetes Care 2003;26:575–581.

25 Nilsson PM, Engstrom G, Hedblad B: The metabolic syndrome and incidence of cardiovascular disease in non-diabetic subjects – a population-based study comparing three different definitions. Diabet Med 2007;24:464–472.

26 Qiao Q: Comparison of different definitions of the metabolic syndrome in relation to cardiovascular mortality in European men and women. Diabetologia 2006;49:2837–2846.

27 Chen HJ, Pan WH: Probable blind spot in the international diabetes Federation definition of metabolic syndrome. Obesity (Silver Spring) 2007;15:1096–1100.
28 Skilton MR, Moulin P, Serusclat A, Nony P, Bonnet F: A comparison of the NCEP-ATPIII, IDF and AHA/NHLBI metabolic syndrome definitions with relation to early carotid atherosclerosis in subjects with hypercholesterolemia or at risk of CVD: evidence for sex-specific differences. Atherosclerosis 2007;190:416–422.
29 Athyros VG, Ganotakis ES, Elisaf MS, Liberopoulos EN, Goudevenos IA, Karagiannis A: Prevalence of vascular disease in metabolic syndrome using three proposed definitions. Int J Cardiol 2007;117:204–210.
30 Monami M, Marchionni N, Masotti G, Mannucci E: IDF and ATP-III definitions of metabolic syndrome in the prediction of all-cause mortality in type 2 diabetic patients. Diabetes Obes Metab 2007;9:350–353.
31 Stern MP, Williams K, Gonzalez-Villalpando C, Hunt KJ, Haffner SM: Does the metabolic syndrome improve identification of individuals at risk of type 2 diabetes and/or cardiovascular disease? Diabetes Care 2004; 27:2676–2681.
32 Pollex RL, Hegele RA: Genetic determinants of the metabolic syndrome. Nat Clin Pract Cardiovasc Med 2006;3:482–489.
33 Chew GT, Gan SK, Watts GF: Revisiting the metabolic syndrome. Med J Aust 2006;185: 445–449.
34 Eckel RH, Grundy SM, Zimmet PZ: The metabolic syndrome. Lancet 2005;365:1415–1428.
35 Clinical Guidelines on the Identification, Evaluation, and Treatment of Overweight and Obesity in Adults – The Evidence Report. National Institutes of Health. Obes Res 1998;6(suppl 2):51S–209S.
36 Lee WJ, Huang MT, Wang W, Lin CM, Chen TC, Lai IR: Effects of obesity surgery on the metabolic syndrome. Arch Surg 2004;139: 1088–1092.
37 Thompson PD, Buchner D, Pina IL, Balady GJ, Williams MA, Marcus BH, Berra K, Blair SN, Costa F, Franklin B, Fletcher GF, Gordon NF, Pate RR, Rodriguez BL, Yancey AK, Wenger NK: Exercise and physical activity in the prevention and treatment of atherosclerotic cardiovascular disease: a statement from the Council on Clinical Cardiology (Subcommittee on Exercise, Rehabilitation, and Prevention) and the Council on Nutrition, Physical Activity, and Metabolism (Subcommittee on Physical Activity). Circulation 2003;107:3109–3116.
38 Tuomilehto J, Lindstrom J, Eriksson JG, Valle TT, Hamalainen H, Ilanne-Parikka P, Keinanen-Kiukaanniemi S, Laakso M, Louheranta A, Rastas M, Salminen V, Uusitupa M: Prevention of type 2 diabetes mellitus by changes in lifestyle among subjects with impaired glucose tolerance. N Engl J Med 2001;344:1343–1350.
39 Knowler WC, Barrett-Connor E, Fowler SE, Hamman RF, Lachin JM, Walker EA, Nathan DM: Reduction in the incidence of type 2 diabetes with lifestyle intervention or metformin. N Engl J Med 2002;346:393–403.
40 Despres JP, Golay A, Sjostrom L: Effects of rimonabant on metabolic risk factors in overweight patients with dyslipidemia. N Engl J Med 2005;353:2121–2134.
41 Liao JK: Effects of statins on 3-hydroxy-3-methylglutaryl coenzyme a reductase inhibition beyond low-density lipoprotein cholesterol. Am J Cardiol 2005;96:24F–33F.
42 Keech A, Simes RJ, Barter P, Best J, Scott R, Taskinen MR, Forder P, Pillai A, Davis T, Glasziou P, Drury P, Kesaniemi YA, Sullivan D, Hunt D, Colman P, d'Emden M, Whiting M, Ehnholm C, Laakso M: Effects of long-term fenofibrate therapy on cardiovascular events in 9795 people with type 2 diabetes mellitus (the FIELD study): randomised controlled trial. Lancet 2005;366:1849–1861.
43 Robins SJ, Rubins HB, Faas FH, Schaefer EJ, Elam MB, Anderson JW, Collins D: Insulin resistance and cardiovascular events with low HDL cholesterol: the Veterans Affairs HDL Intervention Trial (VA-HIT). Diabetes Care 2003;26:1513–1517.
44 Athyros VG, Mikhailidis DP, Papageorgiou AA, Didangelos TP, Peletidou A, Kleta D, Karagiannis A, Kakafika AI, Tziomalos K, Elisaf M: Targeting vascular risk in patients with metabolic syndrome but without diabetes. Metabolism 2005;54:1065–1074.
45 Chobanian AV, Bakris GL, Black HR, Cushman WC, Green LA, Izzo JL, Jr, Jones DW, Materson BJ, Oparil S, Wright JT Jr, Roccella EJ: Seventh report of the Joint National Committee on Prevention, Detection, Evaluation, and Treatment of High Blood Pressure. Hypertension 2003;42:1206–1252.
46 Tight blood pressure control and risk of macrovascular and microvascular complications in type 2 diabetes: UKPDS 38. UK Prospective Diabetes Study Group. BMJ 1998;317: 703–713.
47 Julius S, Majahalme S, Palatini P: Antihypertensive treatment of patients with diabetes and hypertension. Am J Hypertens 2001;14: 310S–316S.
48 Buchanan TA, Xiang AH, Peters RK, Kjos SL, Marroquin A, Goico J, Ochoa C, Tan S, Berkowitz K, Hodis HN, Azen SP: Preservation of pancreatic beta-cell function and prevention of type 2 diabetes by pharmacological treatment of insulin resistance in high-risk Hispanic women. Diabetes 2002; 51:2796–2803.
49 Chiasson JL: Acarbose for the prevention of diabetes, hypertension, and cardiovascular disease in subjects with impaired glucose tolerance: the Study to Prevent Non-Insulin-Dependent Diabetes Mellitus (STOP-NIDDM) Trial. Endocr Pract 2006;12(suppl 1): 25–30.
50 Ajjan RA, Grant PJ: Cardiovascular disease prevention in patients with type 2 diabetes: the role of oral anti-diabetic agents. Diab Vasc Dis Res 2006;3:147–158.
51 Pearson TA, Blair SN, Daniels SR, Eckel RH, Fair JM, Fortmann SP, Franklin BA, Goldstein LB, Greenland P, Grundy SM, Hong Y, Miller NH, Lauer RM, Ockene IS, Sacco RL, Sallis JF Jr, Smith SC Jr, Stone NJ, Taubert KA: AHA Guidelines for Primary Prevention of Cardiovascular Disease and Stroke: 2002 Update: Consensus Panel Guide to Comprehensive Risk Reduction for Adult Patients Without Coronary or Other Atherosclerotic Vascular Diseases. American Heart Association Science Advisory and Coordinating Committee. Circulation 2002; 106:388–391.
52 Ridker PM, Rifai N, Rose L, Buring JE, Cook NR: Comparison of C-reactive protein and low-density lipoprotein cholesterol levels in the prediction of first cardiovascular events. N Engl J Med 2002;347:1557–1565.
53 Ridker PM, Buring JE, Cook NR, Rifai N: C-reactive protein, the metabolic syndrome, and risk of incident cardiovascular events: an 8-year follow-up of 14 719 initially healthy American women. Circulation 2003;107: 391–397.
54 Lee WY, Park JS, Noh SY, Rhee EJ, Sung KC, Kim BS, Kang JH, Kim SW, Lee MH, Park JR: C-reactive protein concentrations are related to insulin resistance and metabolic syndrome as defined by the ATP III report. Int J Cardiol 2004;97:101–106.
55 Yudkin JS, Stehouwer CD, Emeis JJ, Coppack SW: C-reactive protein in healthy subjects: associations with obesity, insulin resistance, and endothelial dysfunction: a potential role for cytokines originating from adipose tissue? Arterioscler Thromb Vasc Biol 1999;19: 972–978.
56 Park HS, Park JY, Yu R: Relationship of obesity and visceral adiposity with serum concentrations of CRP, TNF-alpha and IL-6. Diabetes Res Clin Pract 2005;69:29–35.
57 Jain MK, Ridker PM: Anti-inflammatory effects of statins: clinical evidence and basic mechanisms. Nat Rev 2005;4:977–987.
58 Okopien B, Krysiak R, Herman ZS: Effects of short-term fenofibrate treatment on circulating markers of inflammation and hemostasis in patients with impaired glucose tolerance. J Clin Endocrinol Metab 2006;91: 1770–1778.
59 Duval C, Chinetti G, Trottein F, Fruchart JC, Staels B: The role of PPARs in atherosclerosis. Trends Mol Med 2002;8:422–430.
60 Blaschke F, Spanheimer R, Khan M, Law RE: Vascular effects of TZDs: new implications. Vasc Pharmacol 2006;45:3–18.
61 Roche HM, Phillips C, Gibney MJ: The metabolic syndrome: the crossroads of diet and genetics. Proc Nutr Soc 2005;64:371–377.

Journal of
Nutrigenetics
and
Nutrigenomics

J Nutrigenet Nutrigenomics 2008;1:109–117
DOI: 10.1159/000112458

Published online: February 20, 2008

Nutritional Determinants of the Metabolic Syndrome

Andrea R. Josse[a, c] David J.A. Jenkins[a–d] Cyril W.C. Kendall[a, d, e]

[a]Clinical Nutrition and Risk Factor Modification Center, [b]Department of Medicine, Division of Endocrinology and Metabolism, St. Michael's Hospital, Departments of [c]Nutritional Sciences and [d]Medicine, Faculty of Medicine, University of Toronto, Toronto, Ont., and [e]College of Pharmacy and Nutrition, University of Saskatchewan, Saskatoon, Sask., Canada

Key Words
Fatty acids, monounsaturated and polyunsaturated · Chronic disease · Carbohydrate foods

Abstract
The metabolic syndrome has attracted interest because of its relevance to major contemporary chronic diseases associated with inactive lifestyles and the abundance of food, both of which have resulted in a way of life which challenges our genetic makeup. Changing the fuel mix by the introduction of more monounsaturated and polyunsaturated fatty acids, a reduction in saturated fatty acids, an increase in fiber, and the use of low glycemic index slow-release carbohydrate foods may make a difference, as will increasing the amount of vegetable protein and plant foods such as nuts, rich in monounsaturated fatty acids and antioxidant systems. Nevertheless, these supportive measures will be overwhelmed in the absence of calorie restriction combined with adequate energy expenditure. This situation appears to be one where the subsidiary solutions are complex and the central issue is simple.

Introduction

There is general agreement that the development of the metabolic syndrome (MetS) could be largely prevented by a general reduction in calorie intake and an increase in energy expenditure. Vulnerable individuals exist including those with genetically determined lipodystrophies [1, 2]; however, for the majority of individuals in Western and Westernized societies who lead lives of overindulgence, the MetS is a likely outcome. Much attention has therefore been given to tinkering at the edges of this problem by endeavoring to alter the nature of the fuel mix, i.e. the proportion of macronutrients. These and other maneuvers or dietary manipulations may have significant benefits, but may be overpowered by excess calorie intake. Studies have suggested that the nature of the fatty acids may be important with monounsaturated fatty acids (MUFAs) and polyunsaturated fatty acids (PUFAs) preferred over saturated fatty acids (SFAs) and trans fatty acids. There is also some evidence that the nature of the carbohydrate, whether rapidly or slowly absorbed, may be an issue, together with the fiber content which may also influence the rate of carbohydrate digestion and absorption [3–5]. Studies have suggested that vegetable proteins such as soy may have benefit [6], and that nuts, which were previously proscribed due to their high fat content, may have advantages [7]. Not surpris-

KARGER
Fax +41 61 306 12 34
E-Mail karger@karger.ch
www.karger.com

1661–6499/08/0013–0109$24.50/0

Accessible online at:
www.karger.com/jnn

David J.A. Jenkins
Department of Nutritional Sciences, Faculty of Medicine
University of Toronto, 150 College Street, Rm. 340
Toronto, Ont. M5S 3E2 (Canada)
Tel. +1 416 978 4752, Fax +1 416 978 5310, E-Mail cyril.kendall@utoronto.ca

ingly, vegetarian diets, relatively high in fiber, vegetable protein and nuts have also been associated with reduced insulin resistance and body weight [7–9]. Finally, exercise has been shown to have advantages for the MetS, even in the absence of significant weight loss [10]. However, it remains to be reemphasized that for the majority of individuals a lifelong adherence to reduced calorie intake [11] and increased physical activity is by far the best guarantee of freedom from the MetS. With these constraints in mind, this review will deal with some of the nutritional changes which have been suggested to reduce features of the MetS.

Very Low-Calorie Diets

Very low-calorie diets were popular in the 1980s and 1990s, initially to enhance rapid weight loss by promoting ketogenesis [12, 13]. These diets were the conceptual model for low-calorie, high-protein diets which have formed the basis for more contemporary treatments of the MetS [14]. They demonstrated that after calorie restriction major improvements were seen in insulin resistance, glycemic control and blood lipids independent of and before there was any significant weight loss [15–17]. Furthermore, their effects were seen to be maintained for a long period after cessation of the diet [15, 18]. Concern, however, was expressed that because of the low-calorie intake required, their use may encourage yo-yo dieting. Furthermore, these diets required close medical supervision especially because of water and electrolyte shifts with the possibility of cardiac arrhythmias in those who are inadequately supervised [19–22].

High-Fat Diets

Studies using an Atkins-like approach (high-fat, low-carbohydrate) were carried out in the early 2000s by Samaha et al. [23] and Foster et al. [24]. Both studies were 12 months in duration, with the initial Samaha study published as a 6-month trial followed by the 1-year data thereafter [25]. Results of both studies showed that after 6 months, the subjects randomized to the high-fat arm reduced their body weight significantly compared to the control, low-fat arm (body weight –5.8 ± 8.6 versus –1.9 ± 4.2 kg and –7.0 ± 6.5 versus –3.2 ± 5.6%, respectively). There were 79 morbidly obese subjects in the Samaha study, with 39% of them having type 2 diabetes and 43% having MetS. At the end of 6 months, all subjects on the high-fat diet demonstrated significant increases in insulin sensitivity. Furthermore, subjects with diabetes had significantly decreased triglycerides and blood glucose, and subjects with MetS showed a reduction in insulin levels [23]. In the follow-up to the Samaha study, where subjects were monitored for 12 months, body weight was shown to steadily decrease in the low-fat diet group but increased slightly in the high-fat diet group. Also, at 1 year, there were no significant differences between groups in glucose levels, insulin sensitivity, and total and low-density lipoprotein cholesterol (LDL-C) levels. Improvements in high-density lipoprotein cholesterol (HDL-C) and reductions in triglycerides remained greater on the high-fat diet, and the subjects with diabetes on the high-fat diet showed greater improvements in baseline adjusted hemoglobin A1c levels [25]. At 1 year in the Foster study, which was conducted in 63 obese men and women, body weight was no longer significantly different between groups, nor were postprandial glucose, insulin levels and insulin sensitivity measures [24]. On the high-fat diet arm, triglycerides were significantly reduced at 3 and 12 months but not at 6 months, and HDL-C remained significantly increased on the high-fat diet from 6 to 12 months [24].

In 2004, a smaller study was published by Sharman et al. [26] where 15 overweight men participated in a randomized crossover trial of 6 weeks duration. Subjects started with either a hypocaloric low-carbohydrate diet (<10% energy from carbohydrate) or a low-fat diet (<30% energy from fat). There were no differences between treatments except for a reduction in LDL-C on the low-fat diet arm [26]. Another study was undertaken by the same research group in which 13 overweight women with normal blood lipid profiles consumed both a low-fat and high-fat hypocaloric diet for 4 weeks in a crossover design. Here, the low-fat diet demonstrated significant reductions in fasting total cholesterol, LDL-C and HDL-C concentrations, and increases in fasting blood glucose, insulin levels and insulin resistance assessed by the homeostasis model assessment of insulin resistance. There were significant reductions on both diets in postprandial lipids, and nonsignificant changes in fasting triglycerides [27]. It is interesting to note that the low-fat diet increased insulin resistance, whereas it was originally thought that low-carbohydrate diets may be responsible for this effect. Perhaps this is a reflection of the patient population or the degree of weight loss.

Recently, the metabolic effects of two low-carbohydrate (ketogenic versus non-ketogenic) diets were assessed. Both diets improved insulin sensitivity, reduced fat mass and decreased body weight to a similar extent, but the ketogenic diet was associated with more reported side effects including loss of vigor and energy level [28]. Another high-fat study in healthy individuals demonstrated that the type of fatty acid consumed may increase the effectiveness of the diet. The diet with 70% PUFA was more effective in inducing ketosis (measured by serum β-hydroxybutyrate), maintaining reduced LDL-C levels and improving insulin sensitivity, rather than the 70% SFA diet, which increased LDL-C [29]. Further evidence for differences in the nature of the fatty acid and insulin resistance comes from an Italian study in which 162 healthy individuals were either given a high SFA or a high MUFA diet for 3 months. This study showed that a high MUFA diet significantly improved insulin sensitivity compared to a high SFA diet. Nevertheless, the benefits of high MUFA disappeared when total fat intake exceeded 38% of total calorie intake [8]. A population-based study of over 800 Japanese Brazilians (mean age 55 years) who had the MetS also supports the fact that different fatty acids have different metabolic effects. MetS in these subjects was associated with higher total fat intakes, but high intakes of linoleic acid showed inverse associations with the MetS [30]. More recently, an assessment of the determinants of the MetS in women in the Framingham study cohort, as part of the Framingham offspring spouse study, who were free of MetS risk factors at baseline, indicated that total calories, SFA and MUFA, alcohol and lower fiber intakes, all increased the risk of abdominal obesity and overall MetS during a 12-year follow-up [31]. It appears that increased calories from fat are one of the drivers of MetS, and that the nature of the fatty acid may play an additional role.

In the last 2 years, there have been several studies comparing more than one popular dietary approach in a single study. Dansinger et al. [32] assessed the Atkins (low-carbohydrate), Zone (macronutrient-balanced), Weight Watchers (calorie restriction) and the Ornish (low-fat) diets to determine their effect on weight loss and heart disease risk factor reduction. At 1 year, each diet produced modest weight loss (range 2.1 [Atkins] to 3.3 kg [Ornish]) and reductions in blood lipids, and insulin levels were associated with weight loss regardless of diet. Also, adherence was uniformly low (Atkins 52%; Zone 65%; Weight Watchers 65%; Ornish 50%) [32]. In 2006, McAuley et al. [33] compared 3 diets (high-fat, high-carbohydrate and high-protein) over 1 year in 93 subjects with insulin resistance. At 6 months, all diets showed similar improvements in the features of the MetS (HDL-C, fasting insulin, waist circumference) with greater weight loss and fat mass loss in the high-protein and high-fat groups. However, at 1 year, the high-fat group had increased triglycerides and greater 2-hour glucose levels, body weight, fat mass and waist circumference than that seen at baseline, with the fat mass and waist circumference also different from the high-protein and high-carbohydrate treatments. Reductions seen by the high-carbohydrate group were more modest and sustained over the year. The authors concluded that both high-protein and high-carbohydrate diets are appropriate for people with insulin resistance, and that their prescription should include advice to avoid high-fat protein foods, and to consume high-fiber, low-glycemic index (GI) carbohydrates [33]. Most recently, Gardner et al. [34] randomized 311 overweight and obese subjects to either the Atkins, Zone, Ornish or LEARN (macronutrient balanced) diets for 2 months, followed by a 10-month follow-up period. Weight loss, the primary outcome, was significantly lower from baseline at 12 months on all diets. The Atkins group had the greatest weight loss, but was not significantly different at 12 months from the Ornish or LEARN groups. Waist–hip ratio, LDL-C, insulin and glucose levels were unaffected. In this study, the Atkins diet had more favorable outcomes for features of the MetS [34]. By 12 months, the Atkins group was consuming 35% of daily energy from carbohydrate.

Carbohydrates

Early on, Himsworth and Scott [35, 36] drew attention to the impairment of glucose tolerance from carbohydrate restriction, and since then, it has been customary to ensure that prior to glucose tolerance testing, individuals have an adequate carbohydrate intake for at least 3 days. Studies of high-carbohydrate high-fiber diets investigated by Anderson et al. [37–43] and Kiehm et al. [44] in the 1970s–1980s demonstrated that diabetics could be treated well with such diets as many subjects were able to reduce their insulin dosages. These diets, however, were also high in fiber. A similar approach was taken by Barnard et al. [45, 46] and Weber et al. [47] together with a largely vegetarian diet in a program designed to improve diabetes control and reduce cardiovascular risk.

One of the earlier trials conducted by Kiehm et al. [44] in 1976 assessed the effects of diets high in carbohydrate (75%) versus a conventional American Diabetes Association diet (43% carbohydrate). Thirteen men with either type 1 (n = 8) or type 2 (n = 5) diabetes participated in this weight-maintaining dietary study. After 2 weeks on the high-carbohydrate diet, all men with type 2 diabetes discontinued their sulfonylureas, and those taking insulin were able to either substantially decrease their dose (n = 1) or stop therapy altogether (n = 4). Furthermore, fasting total cholesterol levels were significantly decreased and serum triglycerides were 15% lower on the higher carbohydrate diet than on the American Diabetes Association diet [44]. A further study was undertaken by Anderson and Ward [42] in 20 lean men receiving insulin therapy on a metabolic ward. After approximately 2 weeks, all patients had lower fasting and 3-hour postprandial glucose levels and were able to reduce their insulin dosages. In the early to mid 1980s, following the success of Anderson's trials, the Pritikin Program [45–47] was created which adopted the same scientific basis and dietary philosophy as Anderson. Barnard et al. [46] demonstrated that the Pritikin Program of diet, exercise and weight management effectively allowed for almost all 60 patients in this study to decrease or stop taking their oral hypoglycemic medications and insulin. Blood lipids were also substantially improved [46]. Another study conducted by this group in elderly subjects with a mean age of 78.7 years indicated improvements in lipid levels and glucose control, and decreases in body weight on the high-carbohydrate Pritikin diet and exercise program [47].

Fiber and Whole Grains

Fiber was postulated by Burkitt and Trowell [48–51] to protect against diabetes development based on their African experience and the changes in milling practices in Britain since the late 19th century. Cohort studies have consistently shown reductions in risk for diabetes and cardiovascular disease (CVD) in those who consumed high-fiber foods and larger amounts of whole grain cereals [52–58]. Controlled trials have also suggested that there may be a benefit for increased fiber in terms of improved glucose tolerance [59–62]. Viscous fibers have been shown to slow the rate of nutrient absorption [63], and this aspect of metabolism has been demonstrated to reduce insulin requirements, possibly offering a reason why high-viscous fiber diets may be effective [64, 65]. Recent studies have shown the benefits of viscous fiber from sources such as Konjac-Mannan in reducing blood lipids and serum fructosamine in individuals with the insulin resistance syndrome [66]. In addition, high-carbohydrate, high-fiber meals appear to improve endothelial function in adults with the MetS [67]. A recent crossover clinical trial by Pereira et al. [68] assessed the effect of whole grains on insulin levels. On the whole grain supplementation arm, fasting insulin levels were reduced by 10% in 11 hyperinsulinemic adults over 6 weeks [68]. Whole grains have also been shown to reduce blood pressure, a further feature of the MetS. Over 5 weeks, a barley-enriched diet (20% energy) was shown to favorably reduce both systolic and diastolic blood pressure in healthy adults [69]. Also, in the Dietary Approaches to Stop Hypertension (DASH) eating plan, which includes advice to consume more whole grain foods, both systolic and diastolic blood pressure were reduced along with other MetS features including a reduction in triglyceride levels and an increase in HDL-C [70].

Whole grains have also been favorably associated with other disease risk factors including a decreased risk of all-cause mortality, diabetes and coronary heart disease in the Atherosclerosis Risk in Communities study and the Framingham Offspring study [71, 72], as well as a decreased body mass index (BMI) and increased insulin sensitivity in adolescents [73]. Furthermore, breakfast cereals containing whole grains have been negatively associated with the incidence of type 2 diabetes [74] and have been shown to decrease body weight [75]; however, in this study, the effect on body weight was no longer apparent after cereal fiber intake was adjusted for.

Glycemic Index and Glycemic Load

There is evidence that the rate of absorption of carbohydrates may influence the glycemic and insulinemic response [76]. Thus, it was shown that if the same amount of glucose was sipped over 180 min as opposed to being taken as a bolus in 5 min, the glycemic response was greatly reduced, the insulin response to slowed absorption was flattened and free fatty acids were suppressed over a 4-hour period [76, 77]. The resulting intravenous glucose tolerance test showed a significantly increased glucose uptake by tissues (K_G) associated with the lower free fatty acid levels and reduced counter-regulatory endocrine response [77]. Although glucose is not a model for starch digestion, it illustrates the potential for the rate of nutrient delivery to impact metabolism or metabolic events related to the MetS. The GI is a method for judging the in vivo rate of digestion of carbohydrate foods [3–5]. Cohort studies using the GI classification have demonstrated an association between the intake of high GI foods or high dietary glycemic load, diabetes [57, 78, 79] and CVD [80, 81]. Cross-sectional studies have also shown an association between low GI diets and high HDL-C [82,

83], and cross-sectional studies and clinical trials have shown low GI diets to reduce blood concentrations of C-reactive protein (CRP) [84, 85]. Refined carbohydrates, in general, including corn syrup [86], fiber-depleted starches and sugars in soft drinks [87] have all been linked to facets of the MetS. Although the debate as to whether the intake of these food components is simply a marker of increased calorie intake in general, is still not entirely clear [88]. Low GI diets, therefore, may be associated with protection from components of the MetS.

Soy and Nuts

Increased soy consumption, as a replacement for red meat in the DASH diet, appeared to reduce features of the MetS including insulin resistance, fasting plasma glucose, and serum C-peptide concentrations [6]. In this study, soy supplementation was also shown to reduce inflammatory biomarkers such as e-selectin, IL-18 and CRP [89].

Nuts have also been credited with reducing components of the MetS, and concerns over major increases in body weight with nut consumption appear to be largely unfounded [90, 91]. This may relate to the fact that a significant portion of the intracellular lipids contained within the nuts are not bioaccessible due to the cell wall structure, thereby increasing fecal fat excretion and decreasing energy intake [92]. In a study by Wien et al. [93], 65 overweight subjects were randomized to two energy-restricted diets with either 84 g almonds/day or increased complex carbohydrates (peas, corn, potato, pasta or rice) for 24 weeks. The almond diet demonstrated significantly greater reductions in MetS risk factors (body weight, waist circumference, fat mass and systolic blood pressure) compared to the complex carbohydrate diet. Both dietary interventions were effective in reducing LDL-C, however HDL-C increased on the complex carbohydrate treatment but not the almond treatment (15 versus –6%, $p = 0.05$) [93]. In other studies, nuts have been shown to improve endothelial function, increase or at least preserve HDL-C and possibly decrease triglycerides [7, 94, 95].

Both soy and nuts (almonds), in randomized clinical trials, have been shown to decrease oxidized LDL-C [95, 96], and almonds decreased serum protein thiol levels, a marker of protein oxidation, postprandially [97]. Oxidative stress has been implicated in the MetS by its association with increased insulin resistance, inflammation and endothelial dysfunction [98]. Therefore, the implementation of dietary strategies, including the consumption of soy and nuts, may help to ameliorate these deleterious risk factors.

Alcohol

Moderate amounts of alcohol consumption appear to benefit heart disease [99, 100] and reduce the risk of diabetes [101–103]. The exact reason is unclear, although moderate alcohol intake has anti-inflammatory effects and may reduce CRP [104, 105]. In addition, alcohol may potentiate hypoglycemia by maintaining reduced levels of pyridine nucleotides in the liver, and so preventing utilization of lactate by the liver for glucogenesis, i.e. alcohol appears to break the Cori cycle [106].

Mechanism

The mechanisms for insulin resistance are likely to be many, however, it appears that excess calories are a major initiating factor. Increased calorie loads, free radical generation, damage to endocrine organs and the steady accumulation of ectopic lipid in muscle and liver remain central features. Through the stimulation of antioxidant systems, the redistribution of fat by peroxisome proliferator-activated receptor agonists and the increase in adiponectin to name a few mechanisms, it may be possible to reverse insulin resistance once established [107, 108]. However, these systems are either likely to be overwhelmed by continued increased consumption in the long-term, or by the stimulation of more deleterious pathways. The favorable solution to the MetS problem remains calorie restriction and increased physical activity. In this respect, the experience of the long-term calorie-restricted cohort recruited through the Calorie Restriction, Optimal Nutrition Society, provides valuable information through an average 6-year study of a hypocaloric diet [11, 109]. Although the dietary data do not give a clear indication of the degree to which calories were restricted, the subjects showed a 14.7% reduction in BMI during their first year on the study, suggestive of a considerable calorie restriction. Over the following 6 years, their BMI seemed relatively stable at 19.5 ± 2.1 versus 20.9 ± 2.4 at 1 year. These individuals had LDL-C levels of 86 mg/dl, HDL-C of 65 mg/dl, systolic blood pressures of 97 mm Hg, diastolic blood pressure of 59 mm Hg, fasting glucose levels of 81 mg/dl, fasting insulin levels of 1.4 mIU/ml and CRP concentrations of 0.3 μg/ml. In short, these 50-year-old participants more closely resembled healthy 20-year-olds, and were significantly different in all respects from age-matched controls and from themselves 6 years previously [11]. Similarly, a study looking at a 6-month calorie restriction on markers of longevity came to the same conclusions on the value of chronic calorie restriction, and also provided evidence of reduced DNA oxidative damage on whole blood cells by the Comet assay [110]. Finally, exercise, which is associated with a longer lifespan and reduced CRP levels over time, may also prime endogenous antioxidant systems including glutathione peroxidase and superoxide dismutase, despite small post-exercise increases in oxidative stress. In a study of 5,209 individuals over the age of 50, men who engaged in moderate and high physical activity had 1.3 and 3.7 years more total life expectancy and 1.1 and 3.2 more years without CVD, respectively, compared with those who maintained a low physical activity level. Women showed similar spectacular results. Few therapeutic procedures can claim this success rate [111].

Conclusion

We conclude that the MetS, which is likely to be one of the chief causes in the future for a foreshortened human lifespan, may be prevented by adopting a more primitive diet and lifestyle pattern. This is in keeping with our genetic makeup which shaped our thrifty genes over millennia, and allowing us to survive during periods of a scarce food supply, and the necessity for vigorous physical activity. We believe that elements of these lifestyle components must be reintroduced into the modern lifestyle. Reducing SFA, consuming more fiber, lowering the GI and increasing vegetable protein may all contribute to the overall goal. These positive benefits might be overwhelmed if calorie intake is not restricted, and calorie output is not increased by physical activity.

Disclosure Statement

David Jenkins has served on the Scientific Advisory Board of Loblaw Brands Ltd., Sanitarium, Herbalife International, Nutritional Fundamentals for Health, Pacific Health Laboratories, Metagenics/MetaProteomics, Bayer Consumer Care, Almond Board of California, California Strawberry Commission, Orafti, Unilever and Solae. David Jenkins and Cyril Kendall have received grants from Barilla, Solae, Unilever, Hain Celestial, Loblaw Brands, Sanitarium, Almond Board of California, International Nut Council, California Strawberry Commission, Orafti, and the Canola and Flax Councils of Canada. David Jenkins and Cyril Kendall have been on the speakers panel for the Almond Board of California.

References

1 Hegele RA, Pollex RL: Genetic and physiological insights into the metabolic syndrome. Am J Physiol Regul Integr Comp Physiol 2005;289:R663–R669.
2 Monajemi H, Stroes E, Hegele RA, Fliers E: Inherited lipodystrophies and the metabolic syndrome. Clin Endocrinol (Oxf) 2007;67: 479–484.
3 Jenkins DJ, Wolever TM, Taylor RH, Barker H, Fielden H, Baldwin JM, Bowling AC, Newman HC, Jenkins AL, Goff DV: Glycemic index of foods: a physiological basis for carbohydrate exchange. Am J Clin Nutr 1981;34:362–366.
4 Jenkins DJ, Ghafari H, Wolever TM, Taylor RH, Jenkins AL, Barker HM, Fielden H, Bowling AC: Relationship between rate of digestion of foods and post-prandial glycaemia. Diabetologia 1982;22:450–455.
5 Englyst KN, Englyst HN, Hudson GJ, Cole TJ, Cummings JH: Rapidly available glucose in foods: an in vitro measurement that reflects the glycemic response. Am J Clin Nutr 1999;69:448–454.
6 Azadbakht L, Kimiagar M, Mehrabi Y, Esmaillzadeh A, Padyab M, Hu FB, Willett WC: Soy inclusion in the diet improves features of the metabolic syndrome: a randomized crossover study in postmenopausal women. Am J Clin Nutr 2007;85:735–741.
7 Coates AM, Howe PR: Edible nuts and metabolic health. Curr Opin Lipidol 2007;18:25–30.
8 Riccardi G, Rivellese AA: Dietary treatment of the metabolic syndrome – the optimal diet. Br J Nutr 2000;83(suppl 1):S143–S148.
9 Barnard ND, Scialli AR, Turner-McGrievy G, Lanou AJ, Glass J: The effects of a low-fat, plant-based dietary intervention on body weight, metabolism, and insulin sensitivity. Am J Med 2005;118:991–997.
10 Gaesser GA: Exercise for prevention and treatment of cardiovascular disease, type 2 diabetes, and metabolic syndrome. Curr Diab Rep 2007;7:14–19.
11 Fontana L, Meyer TE, Klein S, Holloszy JO: Long-term calorie restriction is highly effective in reducing the risk for atherosclerosis in humans. Proc Natl Acad Sci USA 2004;101: 6659–6663.
12 Weck M, Hanefeld M, Schollberg K: Effects of VLCD in obese NIDDM (non-insulin dependent diabetes) on glucose, insulin and C-peptide dynamics. Int J Obes 1989;13(suppl 2):159–160.
13 Hanefeld M, Weck M: Very low calorie diet therapy in obese non-insulin dependent diabetes patients. Int J Obes 1989;13(suppl 2): 33–37.
14 Gilden Tsai A, Wadden TA: The evolution of very-low-calorie diets: an update and meta-analysis. Obesity (Silver Spring) 2006;14: 1283–1293.
15 Dhindsa P, Scott AR, Donnelly R: Metabolic and cardiovascular effects of very-low-calorie diet therapy in obese patients with Type 2 diabetes in secondary failure: outcomes after 1 year. Diabet Med 2003;20:319–324.

16 Willi SM, Martin K, Datko FM, Brant BP: Treatment of type 2 diabetes in childhood using a very-low-calorie diet. Diabetes Care 2004;27:348–353.
17 Capstick F, Brooks BA, Burns CM, Zilkens RR, Steinbeck KS, Yue DK: Very low calorie diet (VLCD): a useful alternative in the treatment of the obese NIDDM patient. Diabetes Res Clin Pract 1997;36:105–111.
18 Anderson JW, Brinkman VL, Hamilton CC: Weight loss and 2-y follow-up for 80 morbidly obese patients treated with intensive very-low-calorie diet and an education program. Am J Clin Nutr 1992;56:244S–246S.
19 Henry RR, Gumbiner B: Benefits and limitations of very-low-calorie diet therapy in obese NIDDM. Diabetes Care 1991;14:802–823.
20 Vinik AI, Wing RR: The good, the bad, and the ugly in diabetic diets. Endocrinol Metab Clin North Am 1992;21:237–279.
21 Nishizawa Y, Koyama H, Shoji T, Tahara H, Hagiwara S, Aratani H, Nakatsuka K, Miki T, Morii H: Altered calcium homeostasis accompanying changes of regional bone mineral during a very-low-calorie diet. Am J Clin Nutr 1992;56:265S–267S.
22 Lockwood DH, Amatruda JM: Very low calorie diets in the management of obesity. Annu Rev Med 1984;35:373–381.
23 Samaha FF, Iqbal N, Seshadri P, Chicano KL, Daily DA, McGrory J, Williams T, Williams M, Gracely EJ, Stern L: A low-carbohydrate as compared with a low-fat diet in severe obesity. N Engl J Med 2003;348:2074–2081.
24 Foster GD, Wyatt HR, Hill JO, McGuckin BG, Brill C, Mohammed BS, Szapary PO, Rader DJ, Edman JS, Klein S: A randomized trial of a low-carbohydrate diet for obesity. N Engl J Med 2003;348:2082–2090.
25 Stern L, Iqbal N, Seshadri P, Chicano KL, Daily DA, McGrory J, Williams M, Gracely EJ, Samaha FF: The effects of low-carbohydrate versus conventional weight loss diets in severely obese adults: one-year follow-up of a randomized trial. Ann Intern Med 2004;140:778–785.
26 Sharman MJ, Gomez AL, Kraemer WJ, Volek JS: Very low-carbohydrate and low-fat diets affect fasting lipids and postprandial lipemia differently in overweight men. J Nutr 2004;134:880–885.
27 Volek JS, Sharman MJ, Gomez AL, DiPasquale C, Roti M, Pumerantz A, Kraemer WJ: Comparison of a very low-carbohydrate and low-fat diet on fasting lipids, LDL subclasses, insulin resistance, and postprandial lipemic responses in overweight women. J Am Coll Nutr 2004;23:177–184.
28 Johnston CS, Tjonn SL, Swan PD, White A, Hutchins H, Sears B: Ketogenic low-carbohydrate diets have no metabolic advantage over nonketogenic low-carbohydrate diets. Am J Clin Nutr 2006;83:1055–1061.
29 Fuehrlein BS, Rutenberg MS, Silver JN, Warren MW, Theriaque DW, Duncan GE, Stacpoole PW, Brantly ML: Differential metabolic effects of saturated versus polyunsaturated fats in ketogenic diets. J Clin Endocrinol Metab 2004;89:1641–1645.
30 Freire RD, Cardoso MA, Gimeno SG, Ferreira SR: Dietary fat is associated with metabolic syndrome in Japanese Brazilians. Diabetes Care 2005;28:1779–1785.
31 Millen BE, Pencina MJ, Kimokoti RW, Zhu L, Meigs JB, Ordovas JM, D'Agostino RB: Nutritional risk and the metabolic syndrome in women: opportunities for preventive intervention from the Framingham Nutrition Study. Am J Clin Nutr 2006;84:434–441.
32 Dansinger ML, Gleason JA, Griffith JL, Selker HP, Schaefer EJ: Comparison of the Atkins, Ornish, Weight Watchers, and Zone diets for weight loss and heart disease risk reduction: a randomized trial. JAMA 2005;293:43–53.
33 McAuley KA, Smith KJ, Taylor RW, McLay RT, Williams SM, Mann JI: Long-term effects of popular dietary approaches on weight loss and features of insulin resistance. Int J Obes (Lond) 2006;30:342–349.
34 Gardner CD, Kiazand A, Alhassan S, Kim S, Stafford RS, Balise RR, Kraemer HC, King AC: Comparison of the Atkins, Zone, Ornish, and LEARN diets for change in weight and related risk factors among overweight premenopausal women: the A TO Z Weight Loss Study: a randomized trial. JAMA 2007;297:969–977.
35 Himsworth HP: Dietetic factors influencing the glucose tolerance and the activity of insulin. J Physiol 1934;81:29–48.
36 Himsworth HP, Scott DB: The relation of the hypophysis to changes in sugar tolerance and insulin sensitivity induced by changes of diet. J Physiol 1938;91:447–458.
37 Anderson JW, Gustafson NJ, Bryant CA, Tietyen-Clark J: Dietary fiber and diabetes: a comprehensive review and practical application. J Am Diet Assoc 1987;87:1189–1197.
38 Anderson JW: High-fibre diets for diabetic and hypertriglyceridemic patients. Can Med Assoc J 1980;123:975–979.
39 Anderson JW: The role of dietary carbohydrate and fiber in the control of diabetes. Adv Intern Med 1980;26:67–96.
40 Anderson JW: Newer approaches to diabetes diets: high-fiber diet. Med Times 1980;108:41–44.
41 Anderson JW, Ward K: Long-term effects of high-carbohydrate, high-fiber diets on glucose and lipid metabolism: a preliminary report on patients with diabetes. Diabetes Care 1978;1:77–82.
42 Anderson JW, Ward K: High-carbohydrate, high-fiber diets for insulin-treated men with diabetes mellitus. Am J Clin Nutr 1979;32:2312–2321.
43 Anderson JW: High carbohydrate, high fiber diets for patients with diabetes. Adv Exp Med Biol 1979;119:263–273.
44 Kiehm TG, Anderson JW, Ward K: Beneficial effects of a high carbohydrate, high fiber diet on hyperglycemic diabetic men. Am J Clin Nutr 1976;29:895–899.
45 Barnard RJ, Massey MR, Cherny S, O'Brien LT, Pritikin N: Long-term use of a high-complex-carbohydrate, high-fiber, low-fat diet and exercise in the treatment of NIDDM patients. Diabetes Care 1983;6:268–273.
46 Barnard RJ, Lattimore L, Holly RG, Cherny S, Pritikin N: Response of non-insulin-dependent diabetic patients to an intensive program of diet and exercise. Diabetes Care 1982;5:370–374.
47 Weber F, Barnard RJ, Roy D: Effects of a high-complex-carbohydrate, low-fat diet and daily exercise on individuals 70 years of age and older. J Gerontol 1983;38:155–161.
48 Burkitt DP, Trowell HC: Nutritional intake, adiposity, and diabetes. Br Med J 1979;1:1083–1084.
49 Burkitt DP: The protective properties of dietary fiber. NC Med J 1981;42:467–471.
50 Burkitt DP: Western diseases and their emergence related to diet. S Afr Med J 1982;61:1013–1015.
51 Burkitt DP, Trowell HC: Dietary fibre and western diseases. Ir Med J 1977;70:272–277.
52 Liu S, Sesso HD, Manson JE, Willett WC, Buring JE: Is intake of breakfast cereals related to total and cause-specific mortality in men? Am J Clin Nutr 2003;77:594–599.
53 Liu S, Buring JE, Sesso HD, Rimm EB, Willett WC, Manson JE: A prospective study of dietary fiber intake and risk of cardiovascular disease among women. J Am Coll Cardiol 2002;39:49–56.
54 Liu S, Manson JE, Stampfer MJ, Hu FB, Giovannucci E, Colditz GA, Hennekens CH, Willett WC: A prospective study of whole-grain intake and risk of type 2 diabetes mellitus in US women. Am J Public Health 2000;90:1409–1415.
55 Liu S, Stampfer MJ, Hu FB, Giovannucci E, Rimm E, Manson JE, Hennekens CH, Willett WC: Whole-grain consumption and risk of coronary heart disease: results from the Nurses' Health Study. Am J Clin Nutr 1999;70:412–419.
56 Jacobs DR Jr, Meyer KA, Kushi LH, Folsom AR: Whole-grain intake may reduce the risk of ischemic heart disease death in postmenopausal women: the Iowa Women's Health Study. Am J Clin Nutr 1998;68:248–257.
57 Meyer KA, Kushi LH, Jacobs DR Jr, Slavin J, Sellers TA, Folsom AR: Carbohydrates, dietary fiber, and incident type 2 diabetes in older women. Am J Clin Nutr 2000;71:921–930.
58 Murtaugh MA, Jacobs DR Jr, Jacob B, Steffen LM, Marquart L: Epidemiological support for the protection of whole grains against diabetes. Proc Nutr Soc 2003;62:143–149.

59 Flammang AM, Kendall DM, Baumgartner CJ, Slagle TD, Choe YS: Effect of a viscous fiber bar on postprandial glycemia in subjects with type 2 diabetes. J Am Coll Nutr 2006;25:409–414.
60 Lindstrom J, Peltonen M, Eriksson JG, Louheranta A, Fogelholm M, Uusitupa M, Tuomilehto J: High-fibre, low-fat diet predicts long-term weight loss and decreased type 2 diabetes risk: the Finnish Diabetes Prevention Study. Diabetologia 2006;49: 912–920.
61 Giacco R, Parillo M, Rivellese AA, Lasorella G, Giacco A, D'Episcopo L, Riccardi G: Long-term dietary treatment with increased amounts of fiber-rich low-glycemic index natural foods improves blood glucose control and reduces the number of hypoglycemic events in type 1 diabetic patients. Diabetes Care 2000;23:1461–1466.
62 Chandalia M, Garg A, Lutjohann D, von Bergmann K, Grundy SM, Brinkley LJ: Beneficial effects of high dietary fiber intake in patients with type 2 diabetes mellitus. N Engl J Med 2000;342:1392–1398.
63 Jenkins DJ, Josse RG, Jenkins AL, Wolever TM, Vuksan V: Implications of altering the rate of carbohydrate absorption from the gastrointestinal tract. Clin Invest Med 1995; 18:296–302.
64 Jenkins DJ, Axelsen M, Kendall CW, Augustin LS, Vuksan V, Smith U: Dietary fibre, lente carbohydrates and the insulin-resistant diseases. Br J Nutr 2000;83(suppl 1):S157–163.
65 Jenkins DJ, Jenkins AL: Nutrition principles and diabetes. A role for 'lente carbohydrate'? Diabetes Care 1995;18:1491–1498.
66 Vuksan V, Sievenpiper JL, Owen R, Swilley JA, Spadafora P, Jenkins DJ, Vidgen E, Brighenti F, Josse RG, Leiter LA, Xu Z, Novokmet R: Beneficial effects of viscous dietary fiber from Konjac-mannan in subjects with the insulin resistance syndrome: results of a controlled metabolic trial. Diabetes Care 2000;23:9–14.
67 Brock DW, Davis CK, Irving BA, Rodriguez J, Barrett EJ, Weltman A, Taylor AG, Gaesser GA: A high-carbohydrate, high-fiber meal improves endothelial function in adults with the metabolic syndrome. Diabetes Care 2006;29:2313–2315.
68 Pereira MA, Jacobs DR Jr, Pins JJ, Raatz SK, Gross MD, Slavin JL, Seaquist ER: Effect of whole grains on insulin sensitivity in overweight hyperinsulinemic adults. Am J Clin Nutr 2002;75:848–855.
69 Behall KM, Scholfield DJ, Hallfrisch J: Whole-grain diets reduce blood pressure in mildly hypercholesterolemic men and women. J Am Diet Assoc 2006;106:1445–1449.
70 Azadbakht L, Mirmiran P, Esmaillzadeh A, Azizi T, Azizi F: Beneficial effects of a Dietary Approaches to Stop Hypertension eating plan on features of the metabolic syndrome. Diabetes Care 2005;28:2823–2831.
71 Steffen LM, Jacobs DR Jr, Stevens J, Shahar E, Carithers T, Folsom AR: Associations of whole-grain, refined-grain, and fruit and vegetable consumption with risks of all-cause mortality and incident coronary artery disease and ischemic stroke: the Atherosclerosis Risk in Communities (ARIC) study. Am J Clin Nutr 2003;78:383–390.
72 McKeown NM, Meigs JB, Liu S, Wilson PW, Jacques PF: Whole-grain intake is favorably associated with metabolic risk factors for type 2 diabetes and cardiovascular disease in the Framingham Offspring Study. Am J Clin Nutr 2002;76:390–398.
73 Steffen LM, Jacobs DR Jr, Murtaugh MA, Moran A, Steinberger J, Hong CP, Sinaiko AR: Whole grain intake is associated with lower body mass and greater insulin sensitivity among adolescents. Am J Epidemiol 2003;158:243–250.
74 Fung TT, Hu FB, Pereira MA, Liu S, Stampfer MJ, Colditz GA, Willett WC: Whole-grain intake and the risk of type 2 diabetes: a prospective study in men. Am J Clin Nutr 2002; 76:535–540.
75 Bazzano LA, Song Y, Bubes V, Good CK, Manson JE, Liu S: Dietary intake of whole and refined grain breakfast cereals and weight gain in men. Obes Res 2005;13:1952–1960.
76 Jenkins DJ, Kendall CW, Augustin LS, Franceschi S, Hamidi M, Marchie A, Jenkins AL, Axelsen M: Glycemic index: overview of implications in health and disease. Am J Clin Nutr 2002;76:266S–273S.
77 Jenkins DJ, Wolever TM, Ocana AM, Vuksan V, Cunnane SC, Jenkins M, Wong GS, Singer W, Bloom SR, Blendis LM, et al: Metabolic effects of reducing rate of glucose ingestion by single bolus versus continuous sipping. Diabetes 1990;39:775–781.
78 Salmeron J, Ascherio A, Rimm EB, Colditz GA, Spiegelman D, Jenkins DJ, Stampfer MJ, Wing AL, Willett WC: Dietary fiber, glycemic load, and risk of NIDDM in men. Diabetes Care 1997;20:545–550.
79 Salmeron J, Manson JE, Stampfer MJ, Colditz GA, Wing AL, Willett WC: Dietary fiber, glycemic load, and risk of non-insulin-dependent diabetes mellitus in women. JAMA 1997;277:472–477.
80 Liu S, Willett WC, Stampfer MJ, Hu FB, Franz M, Sampson L, Hennekens CH, Manson JE: A prospective study of dietary glycemic load, carbohydrate intake, and risk of coronary heart disease in US women. Am J Clin Nutr 2000;71:1455–1461.
81 van Dam RM, Visscher AW, Feskens EJ, Verhoef P, Kromhout D: Dietary glycemic index in relation to metabolic risk factors and incidence of coronary heart disease: the Zutphen Elderly Study. Eur J Clin Nutr 2000;54:726–731.
82 Frost G, Leeds AA, Dore CJ, Madeiros S, Brading S, Dornhorst A: Glycaemic index as a determinant of serum HDL-cholesterol concentration. Lancet 1999;353:1045–1048.
83 Ford ES, Liu S: Glycemic index and serum high-density lipoprotein cholesterol concentration among us adults. Arch Intern Med 2001;161:572–576.
84 Wolever TMS, Chiasson JL, Josse RG, Leiter LA, Maheux P, Rabasa-Lhoret R, Rodger NW, Ryan EA: Effect of modifying source or amount of carbohydrate on glucose and lipid control in type 2 diabetes (abstract). Can J Diabetes 2004;28:294.
85 Pereira MA, Swain J, Goldfine AB, Rifai N, Ludwig DS: Effects of a low-glycemic load diet on resting energy expenditure and heart disease risk factors during weight loss. JAMA 2004;292:2482–2490.
86 Gross LS, Li L, Ford ES, Liu S: Increased consumption of refined carbohydrates and the epidemic of type 2 diabetes in the United States: an ecologic assessment. Am J Clin Nutr 2004;79:774–779.
87 Schulze MB, Manson JE, Ludwig DS, Colditz GA, Stampfer MJ, Willett WC, Hu FB: Sugar-sweetened beverages, weight gain, and incidence of type 2 diabetes in young and middle-aged women. JAMA 2004;292:927–934.
88 Jenkins DJ, Kendall CW, Marchie A, Augustin LS: Too much sugar, too much carbohydrate, or just too much? Am J Clin Nutr 2004; 79:711–712.
89 Azadbakht L, Kimiagar M, Mehrabi Y, Esmaillzadeh A, Hu FB, Willett WC: Soy consumption, markers of inflammation, and endothelial function: a cross-over study in postmenopausal women with the metabolic syndrome. Diabetes Care 2007;30:967–973.
90 Sabate J: Nut consumption and body weight. Am J Clin Nutr 2003;78:647S–650S.
91 Bes-Rastrollo M, Sabate J, Gomez-Gracia E, Alonso A, Martinez JA, Martinez-Gonzalez MA: Nut consumption and weight gain in a Mediterranean cohort: the SUN study. Obesity (Silver Spring) 2007;15:107–116.
92 Ellis PR, Kendall CW, Ren Y, Parker C, Pacy JF, Waldron KW, Jenkins DJ: Role of cell walls in the bioaccessibility of lipids in almond seeds. Am J Clin Nutr 2004;80:604–613.
93 Wien MA, Sabate JM, Ikle DN, Cole SE, Kandeel FR: Almonds vs complex carbohydrates in a weight reduction program. Int J Obes Relat Metab Disord 2003;27:1365–1372.
94 Kris-Etherton PM, Yu-Poth S, Sabate J, Ratcliffe HE, Zhao G, Etherton TD: Nuts and their bioactive constituents: effects on serum lipids and other factors that affect disease risk. Am J Clin Nutr 1999;70:504S–511S.
95 Jenkins DJ, Kendall CW, Marchie A, Parker TL, Connelly PW, Qian W, Haight JS, Faulkner D, Vidgen E, Lapsley KG, Spiller GA: Dose response of almonds on coronary heart disease risk factors: blood lipids, oxidized low-density lipoproteins, lipoprotein(a), homocysteine, and pulmonary nitric oxide: a randomized, controlled, crossover trial. Circulation 2002;106:1327–1332.

96 Jenkins DJ, Kendall CW, Jackson CJ, Connelly PW, Parker T, Faulkner D, Vidgen E, Cunnane SC, Leiter LA, Josse RG: Effects of high- and low-isoflavone soyfoods on blood lipids, oxidized LDL, homocysteine, and blood pressure in hyperlipidemic men and women. Am J Clin Nutr 2002;76:365–372.
97 Jenkins DJ, Kendall CW, Josse AR, Salvatore S, Brighenti F, Augustin LS, Ellis PR, Vidgen E, Rao AV: Almonds decrease postprandial glycemia, insulinemia, and oxidative damage in healthy individuals. J Nutr 2006;136:2987–2992.
98 Esposito K, Ciotola M, Schisano B, Misso L, Giannetti G, Ceriello A, Giugliano D: Oxidative stress in the metabolic syndrome. J Endocrinol Invest 2006;29:791–795.
99 Rimm EB, Moats C: Alcohol and coronary heart disease: drinking patterns and mediators of effect. Ann Epidemiol 2007;17:S3–S7.
100 Mukamal KJ, Chiuve SE, Rimm EB: Alcohol consumption and risk for coronary heart disease in men with healthy lifestyles. Arch Intern Med 2006;166:2145–2150.
101 Wannamethee SG, Camargo CA Jr, Manson JE, Willett WC, Rimm EB: Alcohol drinking patterns and risk of type 2 diabetes mellitus among younger women. Arch Intern Med 2003;163:1329–1336.
102 Conigrave KM, Hu BF, Camargo CA Jr, Stampfer MJ, Willett WC, Rimm EB: A prospective study of drinking patterns in relation to risk of type 2 diabetes among men. Diabetes 2001;50:2390–2395.
103 Ajani UA, Hennekens CH, Spelsberg A, Manson JE: Alcohol consumption and risk of type 2 diabetes mellitus among US male physicians. Arch Intern Med 2000;160: 1025–1030.
104 Pai JK, Hankinson SE, Thadhani R, Rifai N, Pischon T, Rimm EB: Moderate alcohol consumption and lower levels of inflammatory markers in US men and women. Atherosclerosis 2006;186:113–120.
105 Volpato S, Pahor M, Ferrucci L, Simonsick EM, Guralnik JM, Kritchevsky SB, Fellin R, Harris TB: Relationship of alcohol intake with inflammatory markers and plasminogen activator inhibitor-1 in well-functioning older adults: the Health, Aging, and Body Composition study. Circulation 2004; 109:607–612.
106 Krebs HA, Cunningham DJ, Stubbs M, Jenkins DJ: Effect of ethanol on postexercise lactacidemia. Isr J Med Sci 1969;5:959–962.
107 Li W, Tonelli J, Kishore P, Owen R, Goodman E, Scherer PE, Hawkins M: Insulin-sensitizing effects of thiazolidinediones are not linked to adiponectin receptor expression in human fat or muscle. Am J Physiol Endocrinol Metab 2007;292:E1301–E1307.
108 Bouskila M, Pajvani UB, Scherer PE: Adiponectin: a relevant player in PPARgamma-agonist-mediated improvements in hepatic insulin sensitivity? Int J Obes (Lond) 2005;29(suppl 1):S17–S23.
109 Meyer TE, Kovacs SJ, Ehsani AA, Klein S, Holloszy JO, Fontana L: Long-term caloric restriction ameliorates the decline in diastolic function in humans. J Am Coll Cardiol 2006;47:398–402.
110 Heilbronn LK, de Jonge L, Frisard MI, DeLany JP, Larson-Meyer DE, Rood J, Nguyen T, Martin CK, Volaufova J, Most MM, Greenway FL, Smith SR, Deutsch WA, Williamson DA, Ravussin E: Effect of 6-month calorie restriction on biomarkers of longevity, metabolic adaptation, and oxidative stress in overweight individuals: a randomized controlled trial. JAMA 2006;295: 1539–1548.
111 Franco OH, de Laet C, Peeters A, Jonker J, Mackenbach J, Nusselder W: Effects of physical activity on life expectancy with cardiovascular disease. Arch Intern Med 2005;165:2355–2360.

Journal of
Nutrigenetics and Nutrigenomics

J Nutrigenet Nutrigenomics 2008;1:118–125
DOI: 10.1159/000112459

Published online: February 20, 2008

Uncloaking the Genetic Determinants of Metabolic Syndrome

Piya Lahiry Rebecca L. Pollex Robert A. Hegele

Robarts Research Institute and University of Western Ontario, London, Ont., Canada

Key Words

Genetics · Polymorphisms · Myocardial infarction · Stroke · Insulin resistance

Abstract

The metabolic syndrome (MetS) is a commonly encountered cluster of clinical phenotypes, including central obesity, hypertension, hyperglycemia, and dyslipidemia. Identifying genetic determinants of MetS will lead to better understanding of its progression and pathogenesis. To further the knowledge of MetS it is important to not only study the candidate genes for each individual component but to also investigate patients with rare monogenic disorders who express a cluster of the phenotypes commonly observed in MetS, however defined. In addition, certain genetic variants have been observed to increase or decrease the risk of developing the entire syndrome. It is apparent that only through complete understanding of the gene–gene, gene–gender and gene–nutrition interactions underlying MetS, will it become possible to determine or minimize the principal complications, namely type 2 diabetes and cardiovascular disease. In this review, we focus on the current evidence for common gene polymorphisms that predispose to or protect from the development of MetS.

Metabolic syndrome (MetS) is defined as a cluster of metabolic risk factors occurring together in a single individual. Depending on the definition used, MetS is predicted to affect >26% of North American adults [1, 2]. This syndrome has drawn considerable interest over the past 6 years since the clustering of these factors increases the risk of cardiovascular disease up to 3-fold, due in part to the associated systemic metabolic, inflammatory and pro-thrombotic disturbances. These pleiotropic deleterious effects promote atherogenesis with arterial plaque formation and instability, which are responsible for clinical events such as myocardial infarction and stroke [3]. In addition, the risk of developing type 2 diabetes in patients with MetS is increased up to 5-fold [4]. Numerous clinical definitions for MetS have been proposed by such organizations as the World Health Organization (WHO), the US National Cholesterol Education Program Adult Treatment Panel III (NCEP ATP III), and the International Diabetes Federation. Each definition uses somewhat different clinical features to diagnose individuals with MetS. However, each definition includes similar attributes such as abdominal obesity, hypertension, fasting hyperglycemia, and dyslipidemia. Furthermore, MetS is considered to be a complex trait because its development depends on environmental factors such as physical inactivity and caloric excess, in addition to sex, ethnicity and numerous genetic factors [1, 5].

There has been considerable debate about whether MetS actually exists as a distinct entity. While it is clear that MetS does not define a disease state, the concept of MetS has proven to be very useful clinically for focusing attention on the excess risk of vascular disease related to central obesity and traditionally overlooked biomarkers such as serum triglycerides [6].

KARGER

Fax +41 61 306 12 34
E-Mail karger@karger.ch
www.karger.com

1661–6499/08/0013–0118$24.50/0

Accessible online at:
www.karger.com/jnn

Robert A. Hegele, MD, FRCPC, FACP
Blackburn Cardiovascular Genetics Laboratory
Robarts Research Institute, 100 Perth Drive, Room 406
London, Ont. N6A 5K8 (Canada)
Tel. +1 519 663 3461, Fax +1 519 663 3037, E-Mail hegele@robarts.ca

Candidate Genes for MetS Components

The key individual components of MetS – abdominal obesity, hypertension, fasting hyperglycemia, and dyslipidemia (defined as increased serum triglyceride and decreased high-density lipoprotein cholesterol) – each have had candidate genes identified. For instance, polymorphisms in adiponectin *(ADIPOQ)* and adiponectin receptors 1 and 2 *(ADIPOR1* and *ADIPOR2)* are associated with traits defined by central obesity [7]. In addition, high blood pressure is linked to variations in angiotensin-converting enzyme 2 *(ACE2)* [8], while polymorphisms in genes encoding apolipoproteins E and C-II (*APOE* and *APOC2*, respectively) are associated with the dyslipidemia component [9]. Study of such genetic associations of individual components of MetS will further the knowledge of the entire syndrome.

Moreover, some gene products may affect more than one defining MetS component due to their influence on common or multiple pathways [1]. For instance, the genes encoding β2- and β3-adrenoceptor, *ADRB2* and *ADRB3* are each associated with both obesity and hypertension [10, 11]. *LMNA*, encoding lamin A and C proteins, has been associated with increased waist circumference and type 2 diabetes [12]. *GNB3*, which encodes the β3 subunit of heterotrimeric G proteins, has been linked to dyslipidemia, insulin resistance, and hypertension [13, 14]. In addition, polymorphisms within genes encoding glycerol kinase *(GCK)* [15] and glucocorticoid receptor *(GR)* [16] have been shown to be associated with MetS, since these candidate genes encode products involved in lipid and carbohydrate metabolism, as well as insulin signaling.

Several genetic associations and linkages with MetS have been reported recently. We herein highlight recent and novel genes that have been evaluated in the MetS complex as a whole.

Insights into MetS from Human Monogenic Diseases

One way to gain more insight into a complex trait, such as MetS, is to study its monogenic analog. For example, familial partial lipodystrophy (FPLD), a rare single-gene disorder that is due to mutations either in the *LMNA* or *PPARG* genes, has been proposed as such a monogenic disease model [17, 18]. *LMNA* encodes nuclear lamin A/C, in which mutations not only result in structural abnormalities of the nuclear envelope, but common polymorphisms have also been demonstrated to be associated with insulin resistance, diabetes, and atherosclerosis [17]. *PPARG*, on the other hand, encodes the peroxisomal proliferator-activated receptor-γ, which is involved in both adipogenesis and energy metabolism, and probably in the downstream complications of atherosclerosis [17]. Because FPLD is progressive and demonstrates the key attributes of MetS, including hyperglycemia, dyslipidemia, and hypertension, FLPD can be a useful monogenic model of MetS [18].

FPLD is characterized by distinct phenotypic stages. The initial stage of FPLD is a gradual redistribution of body fat [18]. This stage is followed by the emergence of dyslipidemia with hypertension [18]. The later stages consist of the development of insulin resistance and eventually atherosclerosis [18]. To prevent vascular disease, treatments are aimed at both improvement of the risk factor profile – i.e. antihypertensive, lipid-lowering and antidiabetic drugs – and newer modalities designed to maintain a balanced distribution of adipose stores [18]. Since MetS probably follows a similar phenotypic evolution, it has been suggested that insights from treatment of FPLD might be translated to common MetS to delay its progression in order to prevent or avert atherogenesis [18]. Understanding the mechanism and phenotypic development of such single-gene disorders is thus not only important for patients with these rare diseases but also potentially for patients with the complex trait of MetS [1].

Approaches for Identifying Genetic Determinants of MetS

Identifying genes for any complex trait, like MetS, involves a range of experimental strategies including positional cloning using genome-wide linkage analysis, genome-wide association analysis, and candidate gene association analysis [1, 19]. Each approach has been attempted with varying degrees of success.

Linkage Studies

Positional cloning involves linkage analysis to map the susceptibility or causative loci based entirely on co-segregation of polymorphic genetic markers within large multi-generation pedigrees. This approach can identify chromosomal regions without any prior knowledge of the disease function or mechanism [19]. For instance, a study involving 250 German families identified a link between MetS and the chromosome loci 1p36.13 [20]. This locus has been previously linked in Mexican Americans with type 2 diabetes [21] while in non-diabetic Mexican Americans this locus was associated with an increase in body size-to-adipose ratio which was estimated using bioelectric impedance analysis [22]. In addition, this locus was linked to lipid abnormalities and hypertension in Australian sibling pairs [23]. A second study that examined 707 subjects from 264 Quebec nuclear pedigrees demonstrated significant linkage for MetS on chromosome 15 [24]. A third study revealed broad regions in chromosome 3, 4q31 and 14p were strongly associated with type 2 diabetes, MetS and cardiovascular disease in a total of 977 Caucasian subjects from 358 families [25]. Finally, a study in African Americans showed evidence of linkage on chromosome 11q24 for lipids and on 13p12 for obesity, whereas a study in Caucasian Americans demonstrated promising candidate loci on chromosome 8p23 for lipids, 14q24 for obesity, and 15q15 for blood pressure [26].

Two general conclusions arise from these linkage studies. First, ethnicity of the pedigrees appears to be a determinant of differences in these putatively linked regions. Second, no specific gene or mutation has been found by these types of studies. Thus, results obtained from using positional cloning must be interpreted carefully especially when linkage studies involve complex traits such as MetS [19]. These conclusions also suggest that replication is essential to increase confidence in the findings.

Genome-Wide Association Studies

Genome-wide association studies are the second approach used to uncover the genetic basis of a complex disease or trait. This analysis is performed without prior assumptions regarding the nature or location of the causative gene. These studies typically involve a large number of individuals and make use of numerous single nucleotide polymorphism (SNP) markers spread across the genome. Patterns of association between the SNP genotypes and disease status are identified and evaluated statistically.

For instance, in 2006 a study reported a novel association between a minor-allele homozygous (CC genotype) SNP (rs7566605) of *INSIG2* and increased body mass index (BMI) [27], while animal studies suggested a role for *INSIG2* in increased plasma triglycerides [28]. Unfortunately, there was a failure to replicate the association between the CC genotype of rs7566605 and obesity in several Caucasian cohorts [29]. This genotype was also not associated with other MetS components, such as plasma triglyceride levels and BMI, in a separate study consisting of Caucasian, Afro-Caribbean and Asian-Indian subjects [30]. These disparities inject a note of caution into the interpretation of genome-wide association studies.

Recently, genome-wide association studies performed in European Caucasians identified a polymorphism within the *FTO* (fat mass and obesity) gene that was associated with both type 2 diabetes ($p = 5 \times 10^{-8}$) [31] and early-onset and severe obesity ($p = 1.67 \times 10^{-26}$) [32]. Future studies in other population groups are required to replicate these associations between *FTO* and obesity, as well as type 2 diabetes. One potential hypothesis would specifically examine the association between *FTO* and MetS, since it has been observed to associate with two of the key components of MetS – obesity and type 2 diabetes.

Although genome-wide association analysis can be a powerful tool to identify disease-causing gene variants, these associations can be relatively weak. The significance levels can be impressive because of the large numbers of study subjects but the actual effect size is relatively small and cannot be tested clinically in a single individual with any meaning or utility for a medical practitioner. Again, such studies must also be validated by numerous replications to avoid false-positive associations due to systemic bias, technical artifacts or population stratification [29].

Candidate-Gene Association Studies

Finally, the candidate-gene approach involves analysis of the association between selected genes within unrelated subjects. This has been a commonly used approach for identifying the genes involved in MetS. Since 2002, there have been at least 16 candidate genes that have been reported [33–49] to be associated with an increased risk of MetS (table 1). Although association studies have been commonly reported, it seems difficult to replicate positive results [19]. For instance, conflicting results of association studies of genetic polymorphisms in *ADRB2* [34, 50], *FABP2* [37, 38, 51], and *GNB3* [52, 53] have been observed. Such disparities may be due to insufficient statistical power, population and phenotypic bias, as well as insufficient sample size [19].

An example of an interesting candidate gene association with MetS involves *IL-6* encoding interleukin-6 (IL-6). IL-6, a cytokine that promotes inflammation and modulates host defense and tissue injury, is produced in activated leukocytes, endothelial cells and adipocytes [39]. In a study of 2,828 Danes, common *IL-6* polymorphisms located in the promoter region, namely –597G>A, 572G>C, and –174G>C, were significantly associated with MetS, according to the WHO definition [40]. Moreover, the *IL-6* –174G>C polymorphism was also strongly associated with MetS in a recent study of 571 Caucasians [39].

Table 1. Association studies showing susceptibility alleles for the metabolic syndrome

Gene	Polymorphism	p value	Sample size (ethnicity)	Definition	Comments
ACE [33]	I/D, intron 16	0.003	1,461 (Chinese)	WHO	
ADRB2 [34]	G16R	0.003	7,808 (Danish)	WHO	Men only
AGT [35]	T174M	0.018	515 (Oji-Cree)	NCEP ATP III	Women only
APOC3 [35, 36]	–455T>C, promoter	0.029 <0.001	515 (Oji-Cree) 122 (Indians, Americans [white, black])	NCEP ATP III NCEP ATP III	Women only
FABP2 [37, 38]	A54T	<0.05 <0.0003	217 (Romanians) 1,500 (Indians)	IDF NCEP ATP III	
IL6 [39, 40]	–174G>C, promoter –597G>A, –572G>C, and –174G>C, promoter	0.007 <0.01	571 (Caucasian) 2,828 (Danish)	WHO WHO	
LDLR [41]	silent SNP, exon 13	0.008	762 (American-Caucasian)	NCEP ATP III	
LRPAP1 [41]	silent SNP, exon 5	0.0003	762 (American-Caucasian)	NCEP ATP III	Women only
NOS3 [42]	haplotype 212	0.01	738 (Spanish)	NCEP ATP III	
PPARG [43]	P12A	0.027	202 (Finnish)	IDF	Men only, see lower SHBG levels
CAPN5 [44]	Haplotype AA-CA (intron 1: rs948976A>G and rs4945140G>A, intron 3: rs2233546C>T and rs2233549G>A)	0.029	606 (Spanish-Caucasian)	NCEP ATP III	
GHRL [45]	L72M	0.02	856 (Amish)	NCEP ATP III	
PC-1 [46]	K121Q	<0.01	130 (Serbian)	NCEP ATP III	Association found in CHD patients
RGS2 [47]	–391C>G, promoter	0.043	2,732 (European-Caucasian)	NCEP ATP III	Men only
CYP11B2 [48]	–344C>T, promoter	0.02	1,540 (European)	IDF	Men only
INS [49]	VNTR I/I genotype, promoter	0.006	320 (Italian)		Obese children and adolescents only

I/D = Insertion/deletion; NCEP ATP III = US National Cholesterol Education Program Adult Treatment Panel III; IDF = International Diabetes Federation; VNTR = variable number of tandem repeats; SHBG = sex-hormone binding globulin; CHD = coronary heart disease.

Another candidate gene associated with MetS, defined by the NCEP ATP III criteria, was *APOC3* encoding apolipoprotein (apo) C-III. Apo C-III is a component of triglyceride-rich lipoprotein particles and inhibits lipoprotein lipase activity. Moreover, the *APOC3* promoter SNP, –455T>C, was associated with MetS in Canadian aboriginal women [35] and also in Caucasians, African Americans, and South Asians [36].

The regulator of G-protein signaling-2, encoded by *RGS2*, has been previously reported be involved in adipocyte differentiation [54] and pancreatic insulin secretion [55]. Recently, a study in 2,732 European Caucasians found that the –391C>G promoter polymorphism of *RGS2* was associated with MetS, defined by NCEP ATP III criteria [47]. Interestingly, this promoter SNP was associated with MetS in men but not in women, suggesting a gender-specific association for this polymorphism.

Another candidate gene association with MetS is *CAPN5*, whose protein product, calpain-5, has been implicated in several cellular functions including apoptosis, intracellular signaling, proliferation and differentiation [44]. In a study of Spanish Caucasians, common polymorphisms in intron 1 (rs948976A>G and rs4945140 G>A) and intron 3 (rs2233546C>T and rs2233549G>A) of *CAPN5* were associated with MetS as defined by NCEP ATP III [44]. More specifically, the AA–CA haplotype was associated with an increased risk of MetS, while the GG–CG haplotype was apparently protective against MetS. The protective haplotype was associated with lower diastolic blood pressure, lower total cholesterol, and lower LDL cholesterol. The association with the overall MetS was likely due to the associations with the individual components.

Table 2. Association studies showing protective alleles in the metabolic syndrome

Gene	Polymorphism (protective haplotype/alleles)	Affected MetS traits (p value)	Sample size (ethnicity)	Comments
AGTR1 [56]	1166A>C, 3′UTR (CC)	1.7 units lower BMI (0.03) 8% lower waist circumference (0.008) 30% lower baseline insulin (0.04) lower fasting glucose (0.08)	378 (UK Caucasians)	Association more significant in men
APOC3 [57]	–641C>A, promoter (CC)	Favorable: Lipoprotein profile (<0.05) Cardiovascular health (0.06) Insulin sensitivity (<0.05) Longevity (0.0007).	687 (Ashkenazi Jewish)	
PPARG [58]	C161T, exon 6 (T_{16} allele carriers)	Higher HDL-C component (0.005)	252 (Koreans)	Women only
PPARD [59]	–87T>C, 5′UTR (CT and CC)	Lower abdominal obesity, dyslipidemia, hypertension, and dysglycemia (0.006)	340 (Quebec Caucasian)	Association with <34.4% fat intake
CAPN5 [44]	Intron 1: rs948976A>G, rs4945140G>A intron 3: rs2233546C>T, rs2233549G>A (GG--CG)	8% lower total cholesterol (0.029) 10.3% lower LDL-C (0.044) 6.1% lower blood-pressure (0.006)	606 (Spanish Caucasian)	
GHRL [45]	R51Q (Q_{51} allele carriers)	15.8% lower prevalence of MetS (0.031)	856 (Amish)	
MTP [60]	I128T (T_{128} allele carriers)	Lower BMI (0.03) Lower waist circumference (0.01) Lower T2D (0.007) Higher glucose metabolism (0.03)	1,286 (German Caucasian)	Association found in men

UTR = Untranslated region; BMI = body mass index; HDL-C = high-density lipoprotein cholesterol; LDL-C = low-density lipoprotein-cholesterol; T2D = type 2 diabetes.

In addition to *CAPN5*, other genes have been reported [44, 45, 56–60] to be associated with a reduced risk of MetS (table 2). One such gene is *GHRL*, encoding ghrelin, a protein that stimulates appetite and regulates energy balance, insulin signaling, and plasma glucose [45]. In a study of *GHRL* polymorphisms in an Amish sample, those with the Q51 allele had a reduced prevalence of MetS relative to R51 homozygotes (3.8 vs. 15.8%, p = 0.031).

A study cohort of 1,286 German Caucasians similarly identified a reduced risk of MetS associated with a variant of the *MTP* gene encoding microsomal triglyceride transfer protein (MTP) [60]. MTP is required for the assembly and secretion of apo B-containing lipoproteins. Male carriers of the I128T polymorphism had lower BMI and waist circumference, less type 2 diabetes and more efficient glucose metabolism as estimated by a standardized oral glucose tolerance test. This protective association was not detected in women, presenting another potential gene–gender interaction for a candidate gene in MetS.

Given that MetS has a complex polygenic nature, multiple factors such as gender and environment plus other unmeasured factors can modulate progression of the phenotype [19]. A recent study has shed light on the importance of diet and genetic interaction. Peroxisome proliferator-activated receptor delta (PPARδ), encoded by *PPARD*, is expressed ubiquitously and has been shown to be involved in the regulation of lipid and lipoprotein metabolism [61, 62]. Within the 5′ untranslated region of the *PPARD* gene, the –87T>C polymorphism was studied in a Caucasian Quebec cohort [59]. Individuals with the –87C allele and a dietary fat intake of <34% of total calories had a lower prevalence of MetS. More specifically, this gene–diet interaction was associated with less obesity, reduced dyslipidemia, less hypertension, and improved fasting glucose levels.

Conclusion

Genetic evidence has been derived from studies done on individual components of MetS and monogenic disease models of MetS, such as FPLD. In addition, it is clear that factors such as obesity, dyslipidemia, hypertension, and dysglycemia are central to our understanding of the progression and pathogenesis of MetS. Thus, by identifying genetic determinants of MetS and its individual components, new pathways may be ascertained leading to early diagnosis and better treatments in the future. In order to study MetS as a whole, approaches such as genome-wide linkage analysis, genome-wide association analysis and candidate gene association analysis have furthered our understanding of this polygenic trait. However, the results of such studies have yet to be applied in a clinical setting and factors such as ethnicity, gender and diet must also be taken into account. Furthermore, the effect of a single gene or polymorphism is likely to be very small and its significance may be difficult to interpret in an individual patient. The etiologic complexity of MetS makes it difficult to obtain consistent results across various study groups. Once such problems have been overcome, it is presumed that diagnosis of MetS at an early stage would diminish the secondary complications of type 2 diabetes and cardiovascular disease before these reach epidemic proportions globally.

Acknowledgments/Disclosure Statement

R.A.H. is a Career Investigator of the Heart and Stroke Foundation of Ontario and holds the Edith Schulich Vinet Canada Research Chair in Human Genetics and the Jacob J. Wolfe Distinguished Medical Research Chair. P.L. was supported by the Heart and Stroke Foundation of Ontario Program Grant (#PRG-5967).

This work was supported by operating grants from the Canadian Institutes of Health Research (#MOP-79533), the Heart and Stroke Foundation of Ontario (#T-6018) and Genome Canada through the Ontario Genomics Institute.

References

1 Pollex RL, Hegele RA: Genetic determinants of the metabolic syndrome. Nat Clin Pract Cardiovasc Med 2006;3:482–489.
2 Eisenmann JC: Secular trends in variables associated with the metabolic syndrome of North American children and adolescents: a review and synthesis. Am J Hum Biol 2003; 15:786–794.
3 Mathieu P, Pibarot P, Despres JP: Metabolic syndrome: the danger signal in atherosclerosis. Vasc Health Risk Manag 2006;2:285–302.
4 Lamarche B, Desroches S: Metabolic syndrome and effects of conjugated linoleic acid in obesity and lipoprotein disorders: the Quebec experience. Am J Clin Nutr 2004; 79(suppl):1149S–1152S.
5 Sale MM, Woods J, Freedman BI: Genetic determinants of the metabolic syndrome. Curr Hypertens Rep 2006;8:16–22.
6 Kahn R, Buse J, Ferrannini E, Stern M: The metabolic syndrome: time for a critical appraisal. Joint statement from the American Diabetes Association and the European Association for the Study of Diabetes. Diabetologia 2005;48:1684–1699.
7 Loos RJ, Ruchat S, Rankinen T, Tremblay A, Perusse L, Bouchard C: Adiponectin and adiponectin receptor gene variants in relation to resting metabolic rate, respiratory quotient, and adiposity-related phenotypes in the Quebec Family Study. Am J Clin Nutr 2007;85:26–34.
8 Fan X, Wang Y, Sun K, Zhang W, Yang X, Wang S, Zhen Y, Wang J, Li W, Han Y, Liu T, Wang X, Chen J, Wu H, Hui R: Polymorphisms of ACE2 gene are associated with essential hypertension and antihypertensive effects of captopril in women. Clin Pharmacol Ther 2007;82:187–196.
9 Yuan G, Al-Shali KZ, Hegele RA: Hypertriglyceridemia: its etiology, effects and treatment. CMAJ 2007;176:1113–1120.
10 Kawaguchi H, Masuo K, Katsuya T, Sugimoto K, Rakugi H, Ogihara T, Tuck ML: beta2- and beta3-adrenoceptor polymorphisms relate to subsequent weight gain and blood pressure elevation in obese normotensive individuals. Hypertens Res 2006;29:951–959.
11 Masuo K, Katsuya T, Fu Y, Rakugi H, Ogihara T, Tuck ML: Beta2- and beta3-adrenergic receptor polymorphisms are related to the onset of weight gain and blood pressure elevation over 5 years. Circulation 2005;111: 3429–3434.
12 Wegner L, Andersen G, Sparso T, Grarup N, Glumer C, Borch-Johnsen K, Jorgensen T, Hansen T, Pedersen O: Common variation in LMNA increases susceptibility to type 2 diabetes and associates with elevated fasting glycemia and estimates of body fat and height in the general population: studies of 7,495 Danish whites. Diabetes 2007;56:694–698.
13 Dzida G, Golon-Siekierska P, Puzniak A, Sobstyl J, Bilan A, Mosiewicz J, Hanzlik J: G-protein beta3 subunit gene C825T polymorphism is associated with arterial hypertension in Polish patients with type 2 diabetes mellitus. Med Sci Monit 2002;8:CR597–CR602.
14 Hayakawa T, Takamura T, Abe T, Kaneko S: Association of the C825T polymorphism of the G-protein beta3 subunit gene with hypertension, obesity, hyperlipidemia, insulin resistance, diabetes, diabetic complications, and diabetic therapies among Japanese. Metabolism 2007;56:44–48.
15 Rahib L, Maclennan NK, Horvath S, Liao JC, Dipple KM: Glycerol kinase deficiency alters expression of genes involved in lipid metabolism, carbohydrate metabolism, and insulin signaling. Eur J Hum Genet 2007;15:646–657.
16 Syed AA, Irving JA, Redfern CP, Hall AG, Unwin NC, White M, Bhopal RS, Weaver JU: Association of glucocorticoid receptor polymorphism A3669G in exon 9beta with reduced central adiposity in women. Obesity (Silver Spring) 2006;14:759–764.
17 Hegele RA: Premature atherosclerosis associated with monogenic insulin resistance. Circulation 2001;103:2225–2229.
18 Hegele RA, Pollex RL: Genetic and physiological insights into the metabolic syndrome. Am J Physiol Regul Integr Comp Physiol 2005;289:R663–R669.

19 Roche HM, Phillips C, Gibney MJ: The metabolic syndrome: the crossroads of diet and genetics. Proc Nutr Soc 2005;64:371–377.
20 Hoffmann K, Mattheisen M, Dahm S, Nurnberg P, Roe C, Johnson J, Cox NJ, Wichmann HE, Wienker TF, Schulze J, Schwarz PE, Lindner TH: A German genome-wide linkage scan for type 2 diabetes supports the existence of a metabolic syndrome locus on chromosome 1p36.13 and a type 2 diabetes locus on chromosome 16p12.2. Diabetologia 2007;50:1418–1422.
21 Puppala S, Dodd GD, Fowler S, Arya R, Schneider J, Farook VS, Granato R, Dyer TD, Almasy L, Jenkinson CP, Diehl AK, Stern MP, Blangero J, Duggirala R: A genomewide search finds major susceptibility loci for gallbladder disease on chromosome 1 in Mexican Americans. Am J Hum Genet 2006; 78:377–392.
22 Cai G, Cole SA, Freeland-Graves JH, MacCluer JW, Blangero J, Comuzzie AG: Principal component for metabolic syndrome risk maps to chromosome 4p in Mexican Americans: the San Antonio Family Heart Study. Hum Biol 2004;76:651–665.
23 Benjafield AV, Wang WY, Speirs HJ, Morris BJ: Genome-wide scan for hypertension in Sydney sibships: the GENIHUSS study. Am J Hypertens 2005;18:828–832.
24 Bosse Y, Despres JP, Chagnon YC, Rice T, Rao DC, Bouchard C, Perusse L, Vohl MC: Quantitative trait locus on 15q for a metabolic syndrome variable derived from factor analysis. Obesity (Silver Spring) 2007;15: 544–550.
25 Bowden DW, Rudock M, Ziegler J, Lehtinen AB, Xu J, Wagenknecht LE, Herrington D, Rich SS, Freedman BI, Carr JJ, Langefeld CD: Coincident linkage of type 2 diabetes, metabolic syndrome, and measures of cardiovascular disease in a genome scan of the diabetes heart study. Diabetes 2006;55:1985–1994.
26 Kraja AT, Hunt SC, Pankow JS, Myers RH, Heiss G, Lewis CE, Rao DC, Province MA: Quantitative trait loci for metabolic syndrome in the Hypertension Genetic Epidemiology Network study. Obes Res 2005;13: 1885–1890.
27 Herbert A, Gerry NP, McQueen MB, Heid IM, Pfeufer A, Illig T, Wichmann HE, Meitinger T, Hunter D, Hu FB, Colditz G, Hinney A, Hebebrand J, Koberwitz K, Zhu X, Cooper R, Ardlie K, Lyon H, Hirschhorn JN, Laird NM, Lenburg ME, Lange C, Christman MF: A common genetic variant is associated with adult and childhood obesity. Science 2006; 312:279–283.
28 Takaishi K, Duplomb L, Wang MY, Li J, Unger RH: Hepatic insig-1 or -2 overexpression reduces lipogenesis in obese Zucker diabetic fatty rats and in fasted/refed normal rats. Proc Natl Acad Sci USA 2004;101:7106–7111.
29 Lyon HN, Emilsson V, Hinney A, Heid IM, Lasky-Su J, Zhu X, Thorleifsson G, Gunnarsdottir S, Walters GB, Thorsteinsdottir U, Kong A, Gulcher J, Nguyen TT, Scherag A, Pfeufer A, Meitinger T, Bronner G, Rief W, Soto-Quiros ME, Avila L, Klanderman B, Raby BA, Silverman EK, Weiss ST, Laird N, Ding X, Groop L, Tuomi T, Isomaa B, Bengtsson K, Butler JL, Cooper RS, Fox CS, O'Donnell CJ, Vollmert C, Celedon JC, Wichmann HE, Hebebrand J, Stefansson K, Lange C, Hirschhorn JN: The association of a SNP upstream of INSIG2 with body mass index is reproduced in several but not all cohorts. PLoS Genet 2007;3:e61.
30 Smith AJ, Cooper JA, Li LK, Humphries SE: INSIG2 gene polymorphism is not associated with obesity in Caucasian, Afro-Caribbean and Indian subjects. Int J Obes (Lond) 2007, in press.
31 Frayling TM, Timpson NJ, Weedon MN, Zeggini E, Freathy RM, Lindgren CM, Perry JR, Elliott KS, Lango H, Rayner NW, Shields B, Harries LW, Barrett JC, Ellard S, Groves CJ, Knight B, Patch AM, Ness AR, Ebrahim S, Lawlor DA, Ring SM, Ben-Shlomo Y, Jarvelin MR, Sovio U, Bennett AJ, Melzer D, Ferrucci L, Loos RJ, Barroso I, Wareham NJ, Karpe F, Owen KR, Cardon LR, Walker M, Hitman GA, Palmer CN, Doney AS, Morris AD, Smith GD, Hattersley AT, McCarthy MI: A common variant in the FTO gene is associated with body mass index and predisposes to childhood and adult obesity. Science 2007;316:889–894.
32 Dina C, Meyre D, Gallina S, Durand E, Korner A, Jacobson P, Carlsson LM, Kiess W, Vatin V, Lecoeur C, Delplanque J, Vaillant E, Pattou F, Ruiz J, Weill J, Levy-Marchal C, Horber F, Potoczna N, Hercberg S, Le Stunff C, Bougneres P, Kovacs P, Marre M, Balkau B, Cauchi S, Chevre JC, Froguel P: Variation in FTO contributes to childhood obesity and severe adult obesity. Nat Genet 2007;39:724–726.
33 Lee YJ, Tsai JC: ACE gene insertion/deletion polymorphism associated with 1998 World Health Organization definition of metabolic syndrome in Chinese type 2 diabetic patients. Diabetes Care 2002;25:1002–1008.
34 Gjesing AP, Andersen G, Burgdorf KS, Borch-Johnsen K, Jorgensen T, Hansen T, Pedersen O: Studies of the associations between functional beta(2)-adrenergic receptor variants and obesity, hypertension and type 2 diabetes in 7,808 white subjects. Diabetologia 2007;50:563–568.
35 Pollex RL, Hanley AJ, Zinman B, Harris SB, Khan HM, Hegele RA: Metabolic syndrome in aboriginal Canadians: prevalence and genetic associations. Atherosclerosis 2006;184: 121–129.
36 Miller M, Rhyne J, Chen H, Beach V, Ericson R, Luthra K, Dwivedi M, Misra A: APOC3 promoter polymorphisms C-482T and T-455C are associated with the metabolic syndrome. Arch Med Res 2007;38:444–451.
37 Csep K, Vitay M, Dudutz G, Rosivall L, Koranyi L: Correlation of FABP2-A54T polymorphism and the metabolic syndrome in Maros County (in Hungarian). Orv Hetil 2007;148:597–602.
38 Vimaleswaran KS, Radha V, Mohan V: Thr54 allele carriers of the Ala54Thr variant of FABP2 gene have associations with metabolic syndrome and hypertriglyceridemia in urban South Indians. Metabolism 2006;55: 1222–1226.
39 Hamid YH, Rose CS, Urhammer SA, Glumer C, Nolsoe R, Kristiansen OP, Mandrup-Poulsen T, Borch-Johnsen K, Jorgensen T, Hansen T, Pedersen O: Variations of the interleukin-6 promoter are associated with features of the metabolic syndrome in Caucasian Danes. Diabetologia 2005;48:251–260.
40 Stephens JW, Hurel SJ, Lowe GD, Rumley A, Humphries SE: Association between plasma IL-6, the IL6 -174G>C gene variant and the metabolic syndrome in type 2 diabetes mellitus. Mol Genet Metab 2007;90:422–428.
41 McCarthy JJ, Meyer J, Moliterno DJ, Newby LK, Rogers WJ, Topol EJ: Evidence for substantial effect modification by gender in a large-scale genetic association study of the metabolic syndrome among coronary heart disease patients. Hum Genet 2003;114:87–98.
42 Gonzalez-Sanchez JL, Martinez-Larrad MT, Saez ME, Zabena C, Martinez-Calatrava MJ, Serrano-Rios M: Endothelial nitric oxide synthase haplotypes are associated with features of metabolic syndrome. Clin Chem 2007;53:91–97.
43 Mousavinasab F, Tahtinen T, Jokelainen J, Koskela P, Vanhala M, Oikarinen J, Laakso M, Keinanen-Kiukaanniemi S: The Pro-12Ala polymorphism of the PPAR gamma 2 gene influences sex hormone-binding globulin level and its relationship to the development of the metabolic syndrome in young Finnish men. Endocrine 2006;30:185–190.
44 Saez ME, Martinez-Larrad MT, Ramirez-Lorca R, Gonzalez-Sanchez JL, Zabena C, Martinez-Calatrava MJ, Gonzalez A, Moron FJ, Ruiz A, Serrano-Rios M: Calpain-5 gene variants are associated with diastolic blood pressure and cholesterol levels. BMC Med Genet 2007;8:1.
45 Steinle NI, Pollin TI, O'Connell JR, Mitchell BD, Shuldiner AR: Variants in the ghrelin gene are associated with metabolic syndrome in the Old Order Amish. J Clin Endocrinol Metab 2005;90:6672–6677.
46 Tasic I, Milojkovic M, Sunder-Plassmann R, Lazarevic G, Tasic NM, Stefanovic V: The association of PC-1 (ENPP1) K121Q polymorphism with metabolic syndrome in patients with coronary heart disease. Clin Chim Acta 2007;377:237–242.

47 Freson K, Stolarz K, Aerts R, Brand E, Brand-Herrmann SM, Kawecka-Jaszcz K, Kuznetsova T, Tikhonoff V, Thijs L, Vermylen J, Staessen JA, Van Geet C: -391 C to G substitution in the regulator of G-protein signalling-2 promoter increases susceptibility to the metabolic syndrome in white European men: consistency between molecular and epidemiological studies. J Hypertens 2007;25:117–125.
48 Russo P, Lauria F, Loguercio M, Barba G, Arnout J, Cappuccio FP, de Lorgeril M, Donati MB, Iacoviello L, Krogh V, van Dongen M, Siani A: -344C/T variant in the promoter of the aldosterone synthase gene (CYP11B2) is associated with metabolic syndrome in men. Am J Hypertens 2007;20:218–222.
49 Santoro N, Cirillo G, Amato A, Luongo C, Raimondo P, D'Aniello A, Perrone L, Miraglia del Giudice E: Insulin gene variable number of tandem repeats (INS VNTR) genotype and metabolic syndrome in childhood obesity. J Clin Endocrinol Metab 2006;91: 4641–4644.
50 Dallongeville J, Helbecque N, Cottel D, Amouyel P, Meirhaeghe A: The Gly16->Arg16 and Gln27->Glu27 polymorphisms of beta2-adrenergic receptor are associated with metabolic syndrome in men. J Clin Endocrinol Metab 2003;88:4862–4866.
51 Erkkila AT, Lindi V, Lehto S, Pyorala K, Laakso M, Uusitupa MI: Variation in the fatty acid binding protein 2 gene is not associated with markers of metabolic syndrome in patients with coronary heart disease. Nutr Metab Cardiovasc Dis 2002;12:53–59.
52 Bagos PG, Elefsinioti AL, Nikolopoulos GK, Hamodrakas SJ: The GNB3 C825T polymorphism and essential hypertension: a meta-analysis of 34 studies including 14,094 cases and 17,760 controls. J Hypertens 2007;25: 487–500.
53 Renner W, Hoffmann MM, Grunbacher G, Winkelmann BR, Boehm BO, Marz W: G-protein beta3 subunit (GNB3) gene polymorphisms and cardiovascular disease: the Ludwigshafen Risk and Cardiovascular Health (LURIC) study. Atherosclerosis 2007; 192:108–112.
54 Nishizuka M, Honda K, Tsuchiya T, Nishihara T, Imagawa M: RGS2 promotes adipocyte differentiation in the presence of ligand for peroxisome proliferator-activated receptor gamma. J Biol Chem 2001;276:29625–29627.
55 Tseng CC, Zhang XY: Role of regulator of G protein signaling in desensitization of the glucose-dependent insulinotropic peptide receptor. Endocrinology 1998;139:4470–4475.
56 Abdollahi MR, Gaunt TR, Syddall HE, Cooper C, Phillips DI, Ye S, Day IN: Angiotensin II type I receptor gene polymorphism: anthropometric and metabolic syndrome traits. J Med Genet 2005;42:396–401.
57 Atzmon G, Rincon M, Schechter CB, Shuldiner AR, Lipton RB, Bergman A, Barzilai N: Lipoprotein genotype and conserved pathway for exceptional longevity in humans. PLoS Biol 2006;4:e113.
58 Rhee EJ, Oh KW, Lee WY, Kim SY, Oh ES, Baek KH, Kang MI, Kim SW: Effects of two common polymorphisms of peroxisome proliferator-activated receptor-gamma gene on metabolic syndrome. Arch Med Res 2006; 37:86–94.
59 Robitaille J, Gaudet D, Perusse L, Vohl MC: Features of the metabolic syndrome are modulated by an interaction between the peroxisome proliferator-activated receptor-delta -87T>C polymorphism and dietary fat in French-Canadians. Int J Obes (Lond) 2007;31:411–417.
60 Rubin D, Helwig U, Pfeuffer M, Schreiber S, Boeing H, Fisher E, Pfeiffer A, Freitag-Wolf S, Foelsch UR, Doering F, Schrezenmeir J: A common functional exon polymorphism in the microsomal triglyceride transfer protein gene is associated with type 2 diabetes, impaired glucose metabolism and insulin levels. J Hum Genet 2006;51:567–574.
61 Oliver WR Jr, Shenk JL, Snaith MR, Russell CS, Plunket KD, Bodkin NL, Lewis MC, Winegar DA, Sznaidman ML, Lambert MH, Xu HE, Sternbach DD, Kliewer SA, Hansen BC, Willson TM: A selective peroxisome proliferator-activated receptor delta agonist promotes reverse cholesterol transport. Proc Natl Acad Sci USA 2001;98:5306–5311.
62 Skogsberg J, Kannisto K, Roshani L, Gagne E, Hamsten A, Larsson C, Ehrenborg E: Characterization of the human peroxisome proliferator activated receptor delta gene and its expression. Int J Mol Med 2000;6:73–81.

Journal of
Nutrigenetics
and
Nutrigenomics

J Nutrigenet Nutrigenomics 2008;1:126–135
DOI: 10.1159/000112460

Published online: February 20, 2008

Dietary Modulators of Peroxisome Proliferator-Activated Receptors: Implications for the Prevention and Treatment of Metabolic Syndrome

Amir J. Guri Raquel Hontecillas Josep Bassaganya-Riera

Laboratory of Nutritional Immunology and Molecular Nutrition, Department of Human Nutrition, Foods and Exercise, Virginia Polytechnic Institute and State University, Blacksburg, Va., USA

Key Words

Obesity · Metabolic syndrome · Peroxisome proliferator-activated receptors · Adipocyte hypertrophy · Insulin resistance

Abstract

In its simplest form, obesity is a state characterized by nutrient overabundance leading to hypertrophy of storage cells in white adipose tissue and the deposition of excess lipids into key metabolic regions, such as skeletal muscle and liver. Ever so steadily, this condition begins to manifest itself as progressive insulin resistance and thus ensues a myriad of other chronic diseases, such as type 2 diabetes, cardiovascular disease, and hypertension, which all fall into the realm of the metabolic syndrome. To offset imbalances in nutrient availability, however, it appears that nature has developed the peroxisome proliferator-activated receptors (PPARs), a family of endogenous lipid sensors that adeptly modulate our rates of macronutrient oxidation and regulate the systemic inflammatory response, which itself is tightly linked to the development of obesity-induced chronic disease. By understanding how PPARs α, δ and γ act jointly to maintain metabolic homeostasis and reduce the chronic inflammation associated with obesity, we may one day discover that the machinery needed to defeat obesity and control the devastating consequences of the metabolic syndrome have been with us the entire time.

Introduction

In the year 2005, 66.2% of Americans were overweight and 32.9% were obese, an increase over the previous 6 years that spanned across all genders, age groups, and ethnicities [1, 2]. Along with the increased prevalence of obesity came a significant rise in the number of individuals diagnosed with metabolic diseases, including cardiovascular disease, type 2 diabetes, atherosclerosis, and hypertension [3]. Over recent years, evidence has indicated that the vast majority of these metabolic diseases are linked to insulin resistance, a condition characterized by the impaired ability to normalize blood glucose levels. There are two major theories behind the role of obesity in promoting insulin resistance; the prevailing theory, known as the free fatty efflux theory, purports the role of free fatty acids (FFAs) accumulating in key metabolic areas, including the liver and skeletal muscle, as being the major cause of insulin resistance [4, 5]. Liver and skeletal muscle are the main sites involved in gluconeogenesis and insulin-stimulated glucose-disposal, respectively. The second theory centers on the inflammatory pathogenesis of insulin resistance and, in particular, the metabolic and physiological changes occurring at white adipose tissue (WAT). WAT, which was once thought of as a passive storage depot, is a tissue becoming increasingly renowned for its innate immune system-like properties.

KARGER

Fax +41 61 306 12 34
E-Mail karger@karger.ch
www.karger.com

1661–6499/08/0013–0126$24.50/0

Accessible online at:
www.karger.com/jnn

Dr. Josep Bassaganya-Riera
Laboratory of Nutritional Immunology and Molecular Nutrition
The Royal Veterinary College, University of London
Royal College Street, London NW 10TU (UK)
E-Mail jriera@rvc.ac.uk

Peroxisome proliferator-activated receptors (PPARs), including PPAR-α, δ, γ, are ligand-induced transcription factors present in high concentrations in metabolic tissues, including liver, skeletal muscle, WAT, and immune cells [6]. All three PPARs are endogenously activated by fatty acids and lipid metabolites [7]. While the individual ligands differ in their specificity and affinity, the ultimate outcome of ligand binding is the induction of PPAR-responsive genes that, among other functions, act to improve systemic insulin sensitivity and reduce inflammation.

Obesity Is Associated with Adipocyte Hypertrophy

One commonality in the divergent theories of insulin resistance pathogenesis is the view that obesity is a problem of supply vs. demand. Essentially, adipocytes, which supply storage for FFAs and triglycerides, cannot be produced at a high enough volume to accommodate the increasing demand to store excess energy, resulting in adipocyte hypertrophy. Hypertrophic adipocytes emit more FFAs and triglycerides than they absorb, leading to the deposition of FFAs into peripheral tissues [5, 8]. In addition to this noted loss of adipocyte function, hypertrophic adipocoytes undergo a significant shift in the types of compounds they secrete. Adiponectin [9], leptin [10], visfatin [11], resistin [12], IL-6 [13], tumor necrosis factor-α (TNF-α) [14], retinol-binding protein-4 [15], and chemokines monocyte chemoattractant protein-1 (MCP-1) [16] and macrophage inflammatory protein-1α [17] are all examples of the diverse set of proteins, known as adipocytokines or adipokines, produced and secreted by adipocytes. Among the adipokines, adiponectin is the among the only known whose secretion is significantly higher in small and normal sized adipocytes when compared to hypertrophic adipocytes. Adiponectin is a potent stimulator of insulin-stimulated glucose disposal in skeletal muscle and an anti-inflammatory agent in the vasculature [18–20]. In fact, the strong association of obesity with hypoadiponectinemia has led some to allege that the downregulation of this adipokine is one of the key initiating steps in the progression of obesity-induced insulin resistance [21]. The remaining adipokines are all increased in WAT during obesity and, as we will come to see, many of them, including resistin, TNF-α, and MCP-1, are pro-inflammatory and negatively effect insulin signaling.

The main factor believed to link adipocyte hypertrophy with the secretion of pro-inflammatory compounds is endoplasmic reticulum (ER) stress [22]. Stress of the ER has been shown to result from a number of factors, including glucose and nutrient deprivation, increased synthesis of secretory proteins, and the presence of unfolded or misfolded proteins in the ER lumen [22]. While the initiating factor in adipocyte hypertrophy-induced ER stress has not been fully elucidated, the cellular response to this phenomenon is a reactionary signal transduction pathway, known as the unfolded protein response, a system designed to maintain ER homeostasis by modulating important signaling pathways [22]. Among the pathways activated by the unfolded protein response in adipocytes are the serine/threonine kinases c-Jun N-terminal kinase (JNK) and inhibitor of nuclear factor-κB (NF-κB) kinase (IKK), which induce the pro-inflammatory transcription factors activator protein-1 and NF-κB, respectively [23].

FFA Efflux Theory of Insulin Resistance

On its surface, the concept of increased FFAs infiltrating peripheral tissues and negatively effecting insulin sensitivity is not altogether complicated. However, there are many facets of this theory which are still unclear. For instance, what are the molecular mechanisms and specific mediators behind lipid-induced insulin resistance? Because of its key role in insulin-stimulated glucose uptake, the mechanisms leading to skeletal muscle insulin resistance have been extensively examined.

Skeletal muscle is a tissue responsible for 80% of systemic glucose disposal whose response to insulin becomes significantly impaired with obesity [24]. In one lipotoxicity model, insulin resistance is caused by the accumulation of non-oxidative lipid intermediates, such as long-chain acyl-CoAs (LC-CoAs), diacylglycerol which is derived from esterification of LC-CoAs, and ceramides. These products can directly suppress the insulin-signaling pathway by promoting several serine kinases, including IKK [25] and protein kinase C [26, 27], that phosphorylate insulin receptor substrate-1 (IRS-1) at serine 307, thereby inhibiting its ability to serve as a substrate for the insulin receptor. Blocking the IKK/NF-κB-signaling pathway, by use of IKK inhibitors acetylsalicylate and parthenolide, completely reversed fatty acid-induced insulin resistance in L6 myotubes [25]. There is also an alternative theory which purports that intermediates of lipid oxidation, such as the ketones, are the main mediators of lipid-induced insulin resistance [28].

Whether or not one believes that oxidative or non-oxidative lipid metabolites induce skeletal muscle insulin resistance, both theories point to some type of dysfunction occurring in the mitochondria [29]. Mitochondrial β-oxidation is a process controlled by regulatory enzymes and end-products of glucose and fatty acid oxidation and synthesis. After fatty acids enter the myocyte through scavenger receptors such as CD36, an acyl-CoA moiety is latched on. In order to be oxidized, fatty acyl-CoAs in the cytosol must enter the mitochondrial outer membrane in a reaction catalyzed by the enzyme carnitine palmitoyltransferase-1 (CPT1) [30].

Control of fatty acid entry into the outer mitochondrial membrane is one of the major sites of regulation. The enzyme acetyl-CoA carboxylase (ACC), which catalyzes an initial step in de novo fatty acid synthesis, inhibits entry of fatty acids into the mitochondria by converting acetyl-CoA to malonyl-CoA, an allosteric inhibitor of CPT1. Thus, molecules which increase or decrease ACC activity significantly impact the rate of β-oxidation. In general, a high glucose or insulin concentration promotes ACC activity while AMP kinase activation inhibits it. It makes physiological sense that high glucose or insulin activates ACC since under such fed conditions one would expect glucose oxidation and fatty acid synthesis to be promoted. The other ACC effector, AMP kinase, is a stress protein activated by exercise that is believed to mediate many of adiponectin's insulin-sensitizing effects [20, 31]. Following entry into the mitochondrial membrane, fatty acylcarnitines transverse the inner mitochondrial membrane through a translocase coupled to CPT2, which then catalyzes the regeneration of fatty acyl-CoA. Unlike CPT1, CPT2 is not inhibited by malonyl-CoA [30]. Once inside the mitochondrial matrix β-oxidation is set to occur.

The complete oxidation of fatty acids not only requires entry into the mitochondrial matrix, but also a concomitant decrease in downstream metabolic pathways such as the tricarboxylic acid cycle. The theory of obesity-induced mitochondrial dysfunction alleges that overcapacitated skeletal muscle mitochondria lose the ability to fully oxidize the high volume of fatty acids, leading to the secretion of both oxidative lipid intermediates and fatty acylcarnitines from the cell [30]. After secretion from the mitochondria, fatty acylcarnitines can then form non-oxidative lipid metabolites such as LC-CoAs, diacylglycerol, and ceramide to activate serine kinases. This incomplete β-oxidation upsets the redox status of the mitochondria by increasing the NADH/NAD ratio, and the departure of fatty acylcarnitines from the mitochondria depletes the availability of free CoAs and carnitines [30]. In support of the concept that obesity is associated with mitochondrial dysfunction in skeletal muscle, it has been demonstrated that the severity of insulin resistance is associated with reduced oxidative enzyme activity in muscle and reduced electron transport chain activity [32, 33]. Thus, while it appears that mitochondrial dysfunction may play a key part in the free fatty efflux theory of insulin resistance, the mechanisms behind this phenomenon have yet to be fully elucidated.

The Inflammatory Pathogenesis of Insulin Resistance and Metabolic Syndrome

Though there is convincing evidence supporting the role of lipids in mediating skeletal muscle insulin resistance, there is equally compelling data demonstrating a tight association between inflammation and insulin resistance. Inflammation is a process principally mediated by immune cells that fights infection and responds to injury. As we have seen, the pathogenesis of obesity-induced inflammation initiates with adipocyte hypertrophy-induced ER stress and the induction of the pro-inflammatory pathways JNK and IKK. The importance of these pathways in mediating insulin sensitivity is apparent in JNK1 and IKKβ knockout mice that are resistant to obesity-induced insulin resistance [34, 35]. Both serine kinases directly and indirectly promote IRS-1 phosphorylation [23]. The indirect serine phosphorylation of IRS-1 is enacted through activator protein-1 and NF-κB-induced production of TNF-α [36].

While adipocyte-induced inflammation appears to be critical in the pathogenesis of insulin resistance, the main inflammatory mediators in WAT are in fact infiltrating bone marrow-derived macrophages, which are initially recruited to the region as monocytes by chemokines from hypertrophic adipocytes [37, 38].

Upon their infiltration and extravasation into WAT, macrophages localize in the stromal-vascular fraction, a region that also encompasses endothelial cells, pre-adipocytes, and lymphocytes [37, 39]. Their localization in the stromal-vascular fraction is highly specific; over 95% of WAT macrophages surround dead adipocytes in what are referred to as 'crown-like structures' [40]. Though their site-specific localization around dead cells is indicative of a debris-clearing function, their pro-inflammatory phenotype exacerbates inflammation. WAT macrophages secrete significantly more pro-inflammatory cytokines and chemokines than their neighboring adipocytes [37], leading to increased levels of macrophages and inflammation. The importance of macrophages as mediators of WAT inflammation and insulin resistance was depicted in mice lacking MCP-1 or its receptor, CC chemokine receptor 2 (CCR2) who, after a period of high-fat feeding, were protected from both obesity-induced insulin resistance and WAT macrophage infiltration [41–43]. There was also a recent publication which demonstrated that IKKβ ablation, specifically in macrophages, significantly enhanced insulin sensitivity in WAT, skeletal muscle, and liver [35].

PPARs Are Endogenous Receptors for Fatty Acids and Lipid Metabolites

As we have seen, obesity is associated with adipocyte hypertrophy, inflammation, and the efflux of FFAs into peripheral tissues. Interestingly, it is these very same FFAs which appear to cause so many difficulties that also serve as ligands for PPARs [44]. Because of the differences in their ligand-binding domains, FFAs and lipid metabolites differ in both their affinities and specificities for PPAR-α, δ, or γ [45]. For instance, polyunsaturated fatty acids, including γ-linoleic acid, α-linolenic acid, eicosapentaenoic acid, and docosahexaenoic acid, all have been shown to bind PPAR-α with specificity greater than the other PPARs [45, 46]. Saturated fatty acids, including palmitic and mystric acids, also induce PPAR activation [45, 47], though their affinities are significantly lower for PPARs than polyunsaturated fatty acids.

One way in which the pool of PPAR ligands is expanded is through enzymatic modification, as adding or eliminating reactive groups, such as a hydroxy or acyl moiety, can have a significant impact on ligand-binding affinity. For instance, modifying arachidonic acid through the enzyme 8-lipoxygenase produces the eicosanoid 8-S-hydroxyeicosatetraenoic acid, which binds PPAR-α with significantly higher affinity than PPAR-γ or PPAR-δ [48]. Alternatively, linoleic acid can be modified by 15-lipoxygenase to produced both 9-hydroxy-octadecadienoic acid and 13-hydroxy-octadecadienois acid, which are both high affinity ligands for PPAR-γ [49, 50]. For PPAR-δ, it appears as though very low-density lipoprotein (LDL)-delivered fatty acids may represent a key source of their endogenous ligands [51], while oxidized LDLs (oxLDLs) activate PPAR-γ [52]. Some questions that are still unanswered, however, concern when, where, and how specific PPAR ligands become produced and under what conditions. As we continue to search for answers, what is pretty clear already is that all PPAR ligands become systemically upregulated in response to obesity. Ultimately, it is the interaction of all these compounds that attempt to offset the metabolic and inflammatory disturbances occurring with obesity.

PPAR-α, γ, and δ Activation Inhibits Adipocyte Hypertrophy

The improvement in systemic insulin sensitivity by PPAR-γ ligands has been used to support both the FFA efflux and inflammatory theories of obesity-induced insulin resistance, with a main reason being that PPAR-γ activation directly inhibits adipocyte hypertrophy. However, it is now becoming apparent that ligands of PPAR-α and δ also have the ability to normalize average adipocyte size.

Approaching the onset of adipocyte hypertrophy as we would approach a problem of supply vs. demand, we see that PPAR-γ ameliorates adipocyte hypertrophy by increasing supply while the other two PPARs reduce demand. PPAR-γ, the most highly expressed PPAR isoform in adipocytes, enhances the lipid-storing capacity of WAT simply by increasing the number and lipid-storing capacity of adipocytes in the subcutaneous region [53]. This task is accomplished by inducing the transcription of genes involved in pre-adipocyte differentiation, fatty acid uptake, and fatty acid transport [53]. In fact, PPAR-γ is required for proper differentiation to occur. The increase in differentiation is mediated in part by positively regulating levels of CCAAT/enhancer binding protein-α, a pleiotropic transcriptional activator that is required for pre-adipocyte differentiation [54]. Increasing the number of insulin-sensitive small adipocytes not only buffers the obesity-induced rise in plasma FFAs and triglycerides, but also can prevent normal-sized adipocytes from becoming hypertrophic pro-inflammatory mediators by expanding the adipocyte pool.

The reduction in lipid-storage demand by PPAR-α and δ is mediated by the enhancement of the body's thermogenic and oxidative capacities. PPAR-α activation increases the expression of the thermogenic, lipolytic protein β3-andrenergic receptor in WAT and brown adipose tissue (BAT) and of mitochondrial uncoupling protein UCP-2 in BAT [55]. Though the effects of PPAR-α activation in white and brown adipocytes are believed to contribute to the reduction in adipocyte hypertrophy, the liver and skeletal muscle contain higher concentrations of PPAR-α [6], and these tissues appear to be the more significant contributors to the effect of endogenous PPAR-α ligands. In hepatocytes, PPAR-α activation upregulates UCP-1 and the expression of a number of proteins involved in β-oxidation, including CPT1 [56], acyl-CoA synthetase, very-long- and medium-chain acyl-CoA dehydrogenases, and 3-ketoacyl-CoA thiolase [57]. PPAR-α also upregulates the transcription of hepatic malonyl-CoA desaturase, an enzyme responsible for catalyzing the reverse reaction of ACC [58], and increases fatty acid oxidation in skeletal muscle [59].

PPAR-δ, like PPAR-α, also reduces the demand to store triglycerides by increasing thermogenesis and oxidation, and, in fact, there appears to be some redundancy in the actions of these two receptors [60, 61]. In skeletal muscle, for instance, knocking out PPAR-α does not have a significant effect on β-oxidation, a response which has been proposed to be mediated by upregulated PPAR-δ [61]. The role of PPAR-δ in adipocytes specifically was elucidated by virally inducing overexpression of PPAR-δ under control of the activator protein-2 promoter in transgenic mice [62]. In response to PPAR-δ overexpression, acyl-CoA oxidase and long-chain acyl-CoA synthase were both significantly increased in BAT [62]; there was also a significant increase in UCP-1 in WAT [62].

While this study indicated PPAR-δ could directly induce thermogenesis in adipocytes, the contribution of adipocytes to the thermogenic response of PPAR-δ ligands appears to be minimal, mainly because PPAR-δ expression in other tissues is significantly by comparison [6]. Skeletal muscle contains PPAR-δ in significantly greater concentrations than the other two PPAR isoforms, and the effects of PPAR-δ in this tissue are quite remarkable. PPAR-δ activation in skeletal muscle shifts the muscle fibers from glycolytic fast-twitch muscles (type II) to oxidative slow-twitch muscles (type I), which preferentially express enzymes that oxidize fatty acids [24, 63]. Amazingly, mice with targeted expression of PPAR-δ also have more physical stamina, exhibited by their ability to run on a treadmill for extended periods when compared to control mice [64]. The shift to a type I phenotype, in addition to promoting fatty acid oxidation, also enhances fatty acid disposal into myocytes [62, 64].

PPARs Differentially Regulate Glucose Utilization

Metabolic disease is not solely a product of impaired glucose uptake and fatty acid metabolism. Rather, it involves a number key dysfunctions occurring in a variety of tissues. For instance, it has been demonstrated that deletion of GLUT4 in adipose tissue induces insulin resistance in liver and skeletal muscle [65]. The organ most responsible for regulating systemic glucose homeostasis and utilization is the liver, though control of glucose metabolism in skeletal muscle is also an important factor.

Since the mid 1960s, it has been known that obesity is associated with dyslipidemia and hepatic steatosis [66]; the greater availability of lipids increases the level of reducing equivalents, glycerol, and ATP, which all promote gluconeogenesis [67]. In the liver, PPAR-α is the most abundantly expressed PPAR isoform [6, 67]. Activation of PPAR-α by its endogenous ligands induces hepatic CPT1 expression among others involved in fatty acid oxidation [56]. The increase in oxidation reduces the production of very LDLs, indirectly decreasing dense LDL numbers and enhancing high-density lipoprotein formation [68, 69]. PPAR-α activation also simultaneously increases hepatic glucose production by inducing glycerol-3-phosphate dehydrogenase, glycerol-3-kinase, and the hepatic glycerol transporters, aquaporin-3 and aquaporin-9 [70]. The favoring of fatty acid over glucose oxidation in the liver by PPAR-α ligands is potentiated in skeletal muscle where PPAR-α and PPAR-δ increase β-oxidation [61].

The increase in hepatic glucose production by PPAR-α is opposed by PPAR-γ activation, a prime example of how PPARs can interplay and regulate each other's actions. PPAR-γ inhibits hepatic glucose production, and thereby promotes glucose oxidation and fatty acid synthesis by downregulating the gluconeogenic enzyme, phosphoenolpyruvate carboxykinase [71, 72]. PPAR-γ also promotes glucose oxidation in skeletal muscle by inhibiting pyruvate dehydrogenase kinase-4 and pyruvate dehydrogenase kinase-2 [73] which phosphorylate and deactivate pyruvate dehydrogenase complex. Although the PPAR-γ concentration in skeletal muscle is significantly lower than either PPAR-α or δ and only 5% of the amount in WAT [74], mice deficient in skeletal muscle PPAR-γ have hepatic insulin resistance [75]. In addition to demonstrating that small even levels of PPAR-γ are necessary in skeletal muscle, these findings further support the idea that metabolic dysfunctions in one tissue can induce insulin resistance in other peripheral tissues.

PPARs and Monocyte Migration

As we have seen, inflammation in WAT, while initially stemming from hypertrophic adipocytes, is perpetuated by the influx of bone marrow-derived macrophages [37, 38]. At the time of the discovery in 2003 that macrophages are strongly associated with obesity-induced inflammation in WAT, it was also shown that PPAR-γ activation significantly reduces the number of macrophages in WAT [37]. At first, the reason for this observation appeared to be related to the effect of PPAR-γ on promoting adipocyte differentiation, whereby reducing the number of hypertrophic adipocytes would indirectly prevent macrophage infiltration. However, as more evidence has come to light, it is becoming increasingly clearer that PPAR-γ, and also PPAR-α and δ, directly impact macrophage migration and function. Monocytes express all three PPARs, and PPAR-γ and PPAR-δ, specifically, are induced during the differentiation of monocytes to macrophages [6, 76].

One indication that PPAR-γ activation directly in macrophages inhibited their infiltration into WAT was the observation that both synthetic and endogenous ligands for PPAR-γ inhibited MCP-1 secretion from subcutaneous and visceral adipose depots taken from obese patients [16]. While this outcome could also be partially attributed to inhibition of adipocyte MCP-1, the amount of MCP-1 secretion from adipocytes in comparison to that of macrophages makes that possibility unlikely. It was also revealed that oxLDLs, which endogenously activate PPAR-γ, significantly inhibit CCR2 protein and mRNA expression in circulating monocytes [52]. Thus, the evidence started to accumulate suggesting that PPAR-γ activation could specifically inhibit the migration of CCR2-expressing macrophages by two different mechanisms, findings which would not only have applicability to obesity-induced WAT macrophage infiltration in which MCP-1 and CCR2 play prominent roles, but also in other inflammatory conditions associated with CCR2+ macrophage infiltration such as atherosclerosis [77]. In fact, upon examining the effect of PPAR-γ deficiency specifically in myeloid cells in mice lacking the LDL receptor (and therefore prone to developing atherosclerosis), researchers found significantly more macrophages in atherosclerotic lesions as well as higher macrophage expression of CCR2 [77]. Perhaps unsurprisingly, it was subsequently discovered that the two promoters of the CCR2 gene (P1 and P2) both contain PPAR-response elements [78].

In addition to the anti-migratory effects of PPAR-γ, there is also evidence suggesting that PPAR-α ligands inhibit macrophage infiltration into WAT by inhibiting MCP-1 production in stromal vascular cells [55]. These findings, however, have only been demonstrated using a pharmacological PPAR-α ligand, which is a significantly more potent agonist than endogenously produced ligands [55]. Therefore, whether or not MCP-1 downregulation occurs regularly with endogenous PPAR-α activation is unclear. Most likely, such an effect would be secondary to the potent oxidative effects of PPAR-α activation in the liver and skeletal muscle.

PPARs, Macrophage Function, and Lipoprotein Metabolism

In addition to being the main pro-inflammatory mediators in WAT, macrophages are involved in the pathogenesis of atherosclerosis, in which they uptake lipids and become foam cells [79], which are among key components of atherosclerotic plaque [80]. Generally speaking, macrophages are functionally characterized by one of two activation phenotypes. In the 'classically activated' phenotype, which we have been mainly discussing thus far, macrophages secrete high levels of pro-inflammatory cytokines and chemokines, including TNF-α and MCP-1 [81]. Conversely, 'alternatively activated' macrophages have a reparative phenotype and secrete immunomodulatory cytokines, such as IL-10 and transforming growth factor-β [81]. Though there is no evidence suggesting that PPAR activation can increase the ratio of 'alternatively activated' to 'classically activated' macrophages, PPAR ligands do appear to play a role in mediating macrophage function by affecting pro-inflammatory cytokine secretion and enhancing reverse cholesterol transport in the vasculature.

In vitro experiments have demonstrated that both endogenous and synthetic agonists of PPAR-γ inhibit lipopolysaccharide-induced macrophage activation [82]. Unlike the effects of PPAR-γ on genes involved in fatty acid metabolism, inhibition of pro-inflammatory genes in macrophages does not involve transcriptional regulation. Rather, the mechanism involves post-translational modification. After ligand binding in the macrophage, the ligand-binding domain of PPAR-γ becomes sumoylated [83]. Sumo is a protein similar to ubiquitin which, upon attachment to a transcription factor, often signals for transcriptional repression. Upon sumoylation, PPAR-γ transmigrates to the nuclear receptor co-repressor-histone deacetylase-3 complexes at pro-inflammatory gene promoters [83]. The presence of PPAR-γ at these sites inhibits the ubiquitination of these co-repressor complexes that is normally induced by lipopolysaccharide treatment, thereby maintaining these pro-inflammatory genes in the repressed state [83]. While this anti-inflammatory of PPAR-γ in macrophages has recently been characterized, there is also evidence suggesting that PPAR-δ mediates many of these effects in PPAR-γ-null macrophages, indicating that there is a built-in redundancy in this response [82].

In addition to modulating pro-inflammatory secretion, PPAR ligands affect macrophage function by enhancing reverse cholesterol transport. The reduced storage capacity of WAT not only increases lipid deposition in peripheral tissues such as skeletal muscle, heart, and liver, but also inhibits uptake of circulating LDLs [84]. The oxidation of LDLs in the vasculature is one of the early steps in the formation of plaque [85]. OxLDLs increase smooth muscle proliferation and promote endothelial cell activation [85], leading to the formation of thrombi. When these clots occur in the coronary or carotid arteries or break loose and become deposited in these regions, myocardial infarctions or strokes are all-to-familiar outcomes. Interestingly, the pro-atherogenic effect of macrophages in the vascular system is very similar to the pro-inflammatory effect in WAT. In atherosclerosis, macrophages are recruited to clear the lipids and cholesterol from oxLDLs but then develop a pro-inflammatory phenotype [86], resulting in increased vascular inflammation and more macrophage infiltration. In fact, mice deficient in MCP-1 or CCR2, just as the case with obesity-induced insulin resistance, are also protected from the development of atherosclerotic plaques [87, 88]. The continuous uptake of lipids by macrophages results in the formation of foam cells, which accumulate along the arterial wall and are among the key components of fatty streaks [79]. Fatty streaks are characterized of layers of foam cells and lipid droplets within the intimal smooth muscle and are the first grossly observable features of a type II atherosclerotic lesion [89].

PPARs exert their anti-atherogenic effects by reducing vascular inflammation and enhancing the clearance of oxLDLs [86, 90]. The uptake of oxLDLs by macrophages is mediated through scavenger receptors CD36, CD68, and scavenger receptor A [86]. Whole-body elimination of CD36, a PPAR-γ-responsive gene, actually provides protection from foam cell development, which would perhaps elude that PPAR-γ is pro-atherogenic [91]. Studies have shown, however, that PPAR-γ is anti-atherogenic; the reason being that simultaneous to the induction of CD36, both PPAR-γ and PPAR-α ligands induce the expression of the nuclear receptor liver X receptor-α [86, 92, 93]. Liver X receptor-α activates genes responsible for reverse cholesterol transport, including ATP-binding cassette transporters, ABCA-1 and ABCG-1, which increase lipid transport to high-density lipoproteins and thereby inhibit foam cell formation [78, 92, 93]. In addition to PPAR-α and γ, there are some reports indicating that PPAR-δ may play a role in promoting reverse cholesterol transport by inducing ABCA-1 [92], but thus far these findings have been inconsistent and PPAR-δ does not appear to be critical for ABCA-1 expression [93].

Conclusions

To classify obesity simply as an inflammatory disease or a disorder in lipid metabolism does not do justice to the amazingly complex nature of this condition. Because the free fatty efflux and inflammatory theories regarding the progression of obesity-induced insulin resistance both have a significant amount of accumulated evidence, it is likely that they will eventually be merged together in a unifying theory of insulin resistance. In this regard, PPARs can be thought of as a link between the two diverging theories, as their systemic integration and cooperation in improving both inflammation and increasing oxidation of excess lipids has made them ideal homeostatic regulators of glucose homeostasis. Learning how PPARs function under different physiological conditions appears to be an ideal step in understanding how nature intended our bodies to cope with the metabolic and inflammatory stresses of obesity.

Disclosure Statement

The authors declare that no financial or other conflict of interest exists in relation to the content of the article.

References

1 Ogden CL, Carroll MD, Curtin LR, McDowell MA, Tabak CJ, Flegal KM: Prevalence of overweight and obesity in the United States, 1999–2004. JAMA 2006;295:1549–1555.
2 Flegal KM, Ogden CL, Carroll MD: Prevalence and trends in overweight in Mexican-American adults and children. Nutr Rev 2004;62:S144–S148.
3 Finkelstein EA, Fiebelkorn IC, Wang G: National medical spending attributable to overweight and obesity: how much, and who's paying? Health Aff (Millwood) 2003;Suppl Web Exclusives:W3-219–226.
4 Lewis GF, Carpentier A, Adeli K, Giacca A: Disordered fat storage and mobilization in the pathogenesis of insulin resistance and type 2 diabetes. Endocr Rev 2002;23:201–229.

5 Groop LC, Saloranta C, Shank M, Bonadonna RC, Ferrannini E, DeFronzo RA: The role of free fatty acid metabolism in the pathogenesis of insulin resistance in obesity and noninsulin-dependent diabetes mellitus. J Clin Endocrinol Metab 1991;72:96–107.
6 Braissant O, Foufelle F, Scotto C, Dauca M, Wahli W: Differential expression of peroxisome proliferator-activated receptors (PPARs): tissue distribution of PPAR-alpha, -beta, and -gamma in the adult rat. Endocrinology 1996;137:354–366.
7 Vidal-Puig AJ, Considine RV, Jimenez-Linan M, Werman A, Pories WJ, Caro JF, Flier JS: Peroxisome proliferator-activated receptor gene expression in human tissues. Effects of obesity, weight loss, and regulation by insulin and glucocorticoids. J Clin Invest 1997; 99:2416–2422.
8 Campbell PJ, Carlson MG, Nurjhan N: Fat metabolism in human obesity. Am J Physiol 1994;266:E600–E605.
9 Hu E, Liang P, Spiegelman BM: AdipoQ is a novel adipose-specific gene dysregulated in obesity. J Biol Chem 1996;271:10697–10703.
10 Maffei M, Fei H, Lee GH, Dani C, Leroy P, Zhang Y, Proenca R, Negrel R, Ailhaud G, Friedman JM: Increased expression in adipocytes of ob RNA in mice with lesions of the hypothalamus and with mutations at the db locus. Proc Natl Acad Sci USA 1995;92:6957–6960.
11 Hug C, Lodish HF: Medicine. Visfatin: a new adipokine. Science 2005;307:366–367.
12 Steppan CM, Bailey ST, Bhat S, Brown EJ, Banerjee RR, Wright CM, Patel HR, Ahima RS, Lazar MA: The hormone resistin links obesity to diabetes. Nature 2001;409:307–312.
13 Bruun JM, Lihn AS, Madan AK, Pedersen SB, Schiott KM, Fain JN, Richelsen B: Higher production of IL-8 in visceral vs. subcutaneous adipose tissue. Implication of nonadipose cells in adipose tissue. Am J Physiol Endocrinol Metab 2004;286:E8–E13.
14 Hotamisligil GS, Shargill NS, Spiegelman BM: Adipose expression of tumor necrosis factor-alpha: direct role in obesity-linked insulin resistance. Science 1993;259:87–91.
15 Cho YM, Youn BS, Lee H, Lee N, Min SS, Kwak SH, Lee HK, Park KS: Plasma retinol-binding protein-4 concentrations are elevated in human subjects with impaired glucose tolerance and type 2 diabetes. Diabetes Care 2006;29:2457–2461.
16 Bruun JM, Lihn AS, Pedersen SB, Richelsen B: Monocyte chemoattractant protein-1 release is higher in visceral than subcutaneous human adipose tissue (AT): implication of macrophages resident in the AT. J Clin Endocrinol Metab 2005;90:2282–2289.
17 Gerhardt CC, Romero IA, Cancello R, Camoin L, Strosberg AD: Chemokines control fat accumulation and leptin secretion by cultured human adipocytes. Mol Cell Endocrinol 2001;175:81–92.
18 Berg AH, Combs TP, Du X, Brownlee M, Scherer PE: The adipocyte-secreted protein Acrp30 enhances hepatic insulin action. Nat Med 2001;7:947–953.
19 Fruebis J, Tsao TS, Javorschi S, Ebbets-Reed D, Erickson MR, Yen FT, Bihain BE, Lodish HF: Proteolytic cleavage product of 30-kDa adipocyte complement-related protein increases fatty acid oxidation in muscle and causes weight loss in mice. Proc Natl Acad Sci USA 2001;98:2005–2010.
20 Yamauchi T, Kamon J, Minokoshi Y, Ito Y, Waki H, Uchida S, Yamashita S, Noda M, Kita S, Ueki K, Eto K, Akanuma Y, Froguel P, Foufelle F, Ferre P, Carling D, Kimura S, Nagai R, Kahn BB, Kadowaki T: Adiponectin stimulates glucose utilization and fatty-acid oxidation by activating AMP-activated protein kinase. Nat Med 2002;8:1288–1295.
21 Matsushita K, Yatsuya H, Tamakoshi K, Wada K, Otsuka R, Takefuji S, Sugiura K, Kondo T, Murohara T, Toyoshima H: Comparison of circulating adiponectin and proinflammatory markers regarding their association with metabolic syndrome in Japanese men. Arterioscler Thromb Vasc Biol 2006; 26:871–876.
22 Ozcan U, Cao Q, Yilmaz E, Lee AH, Iwakoshi NN, Ozdelen E, Tuncman G, Gorgun C, Glimcher LH, Hotamisligil GS: Endoplasmic reticulum stress links obesity, insulin action, and type 2 diabetes. Science 2004;306:457–461.
23 Wellen KE, Hotamisligil GS: Inflammation, stress, and diabetes. J Clin Invest 2005;115: 1111–1119.
24 Barish GD, Narkar VA, Evans RM: PPAR delta: a dagger in the heart of the metabolic syndrome. J Clin Invest 2006;116:590–597.
25 Sinha S, Perdomo G, Brown NF, O'Doherty RM: Fatty acid-induced insulin resistance in L6 myotubes is prevented by inhibition of activation and nuclear localization of nuclear factor kappa B. J Biol Chem 2004;279:41294–41301.
26 Seifert R, Schachtele C, Schultz G: Activation of protein kinase C by cis-and trans-octadecadienoic acids in intact human platelets and its potentiation by diacylglycerol. Biochem Biophys Res Commun 1987;149:762–768.
27 Danielsen AG, Liu F, Hosomi Y, Shii K, Roth RA: Activation of protein kinase C alpha inhibits signaling by members of the insulin receptor family. J Biol Chem 1995;270: 21600–21605.
28 An J, Muoio DM, Shiota M, Fujimoto Y, Cline GW, Shulman GI, Koves TR, Stevens R, Millington D, Newgard CB: Hepatic expression of malonyl-CoA decarboxylase reverses muscle, liver and whole-animal insulin resistance. Nat Med 2004;10:268–274.
29 Lowell BB, Shulman GI: Mitochondrial dysfunction and type 2 diabetes. Science 2005; 307:384–387.
30 Muoio DM, Newgard CB: Obesity-related derangements in metabolic regulation. Annu Rev Biochem 2006;75:367–401.
31 Ouchi N, Kihara S, Arita Y, Okamoto Y, Maeda K, Kuriyama H, Hotta K, Nishida M, Takahashi M, Muraguchi M, Ohmoto Y, Nakamura T, Yamashita S, Funahashi T, Matsuzawa Y: Adiponectin, an adipocyte-derived plasma protein, inhibits endothelial NF-kappaB signaling through a cAMP-dependent pathway. Circulation 2000;102:1296–1301.
32 Kelley DE, He J, Menshikova EV, Ritov VB: Dysfunction of mitochondria in human skeletal muscle in type 2 diabetes. Diabetes 2002;51:2944–2950.
33 Ritov VB, Menshikova EV, He J, Ferrell RE, Goodpaster BH, Kelley DE: Deficiency of subsarcolemmal mitochondria in obesity and type 2 diabetes. Diabetes 2005;54:8–14.
34 Hirosumi J, Tuncman G, Chang L, Gorgun CZ, Uysal KT, Maeda K, Karin M, Hotamisligil GS: A central role for JNK in obesity and insulin resistance. Nature 2002;420:333–336.
35 Arkan MC, Hevener AL, Greten FR, Maeda S, Li ZW, Long JM, Wynshaw-Boris A, Poli G, Olefsky J, Karin M: IKK-beta links inflammation to obesity-induced insulin resistance. Nat Med 2005;11:191–198.
36 Gao Z, Hwang D, Bataille F, Lefevre M, York D, Quon MJ, Ye J: Serine phosphorylation of insulin receptor substrate 1 by inhibitor kappa B kinase complex. J Biol Chem 2002;77: 48115–48121.
37 Weisberg SP, McCann D, Desai M, Rosenbaum M, Leibel RL, Ferrante AW Jr: Obesity is associated with macrophage accumulation in adipose tissue. J Clin Invest 2003;112: 1796–1808.
38 Xu H, Barnes GT, Yang Q, Tan G, Yang D, Chou CJ, Sole J, Nichols A, Ross JS, Tartaglia LA, Chen H: Chronic inflammation in fat plays a crucial role in the development of obesity-related insulin resistance. J Clin Invest 2003;112:1821–1830.
39 Robker RL, Collins RG, Beaudet AL, Mersmann HJ, Smith CW: Leukocyte migration in adipose tissue of mice null for ICAM-1 and Mac-1 adhesion receptors. Obes Res 2004;12:936–940.
40 Cinti S, Mitchell G, Barbatelli G, Murano I, Ceresi E, Faloia E, Wang S, Fortier M, Greenberg AS, Obin MS: Adipocyte death defines macrophage localization and function in adipose tissue of obese mice and humans. J Lipid Res 2005;46:2347–2355.
41 Weisberg SP, Hunter D, Huber R, Lemieux J, Slaymaker S, Vaddi K, Charo I, Leibel RL, Ferrante AW Jr: CCR2 modulates inflammatory and metabolic effects of high-fat feeding. J Clin Invest 2006;116:115–124.

42 Kanda H, Tateya S, Tamori Y, Kotani K, Hiasa K, Kitazawa R, Kitazawa S, Miyachi H, Maeda S, Egashira K, Kasuga M: MCP-1 contributes to macrophage infiltration into adipose tissue, insulin resistance, and hepatic steatosis in obesity. J Clin Invest 2006;116: 1494–1505.
43 Kamei N, Tobe K, Suzuki R, Ohsugi M, Watanabe T, Kubota N, Ohtsuka-Kowatari N, Kumagai K, Sakamoto K, Kobayashi M, Yamauchi T, Ueki K, Oishi Y, Nishimura S, Manabe I, Hashimoto H, Ohnishi Y, Ogata H, Tokuyama K, Tsunoda M, Ide T, Murakami K, Nagai R, Kadowaki T: Overexpression of monocyte chemoattractant protein-1 in adipose tissues causes macrophage recruitment and insulin resistance. J Biol Chem 2006;281:26602–26614.
44 Guri A, Hontecillas R, Bassaganya-Riera J: Peroxisome proliferator-activated receptors: bridging metabolic syndrome with molecular nutrition. Clin Nutr 2006;25:871–885.
45 Desvergne B, Wahli W: Peroxisome proliferator-activated receptors: nuclear control of metabolism. Endocr Rev 1999;20:649–688.
46 Willson TM, Wahli W: Peroxisome proliferator-activated receptor agonists. Curr Opin Chem Biol 1997;1:235–241.
47 Banner CD, Gottlicher M, Widmark E, Sjovall J, Rafter JJ, Gustafsson JA: A systematic analytical chemistry/cell assay approach to isolate activators of orphan nuclear receptors from biological extracts: characterization of peroxisome proliferator-activated receptor activators in plasma. J Lipid Res 1993;34: 1583–1591.
48 Muga SJ, Thuillier P, Pavone A, Rundhaug JE, Boeglin WE, Jisaka M, Brash AR, Fischer SM: 8S-lipoxygenase products activate peroxisome proliferator-activated receptor alpha and induce differentiation in murine keratinocytes. Cell Growth Differ 2000;11: 447–454.
49 Nagy L, Tontonoz P, Alvarez JG, Chen H, Evans RM: Oxidized LDL regulates macrophage gene expression through ligand activation of PPARgamma. Cell 1998;93:229–240.
50 Forman BM, Tontonoz P, Chen J, Brun RP, Spiegelman BM, Evans RM: 15-Deoxy-delta 12, 14-prostaglandin J2 is a ligand for the adipocyte determination factor PPAR gamma. Cell 1995;83:803–812.
51 Chawla A, Lee CH, Barak Y, He W, Rosenfeld J, Liao D, Han J, Kang H, Evans RM: PPARdelta is a very low-density lipoprotein sensor in macrophages. Proc Natl Acad Sci USA 2003; 100:1268–1273.
52 Han KH, Chang MK, Boullier A, Green SR, Li A, Glass CK, Quehenberger O: Oxidized LDL reduces monocyte CCR2 expression through pathways involving peroxisome proliferator-activated receptor gamma. J Clin Invest 2000;106:793–802.
53 Tontonoz P, Hu E, Spiegelman BM: Regulation of adipocyte gene expression and differentiation by peroxisome proliferator activated receptor gamma. Curr Opin Genet Dev 1995;5:571–576.
54 Otto TC, Lane MD: Adipose development: from stem cell to adipocyte. Crit Rev Biochem Mol Biol 2005;40:229–242.
55 Tsuchida A, Yamauchi T, Takekawa S, Hada Y, Ito Y, Maki T, Kadowaki T: Peroxisome proliferator-activated receptor (PPAR)alpha activation increases adiponectin receptors and reduces obesity-related inflammation in adipose tissue: comparison of activation of PPARalpha, PPARgamma, and their combination. Diabetes 2005;54:3358–3370.
56 Nagasawa T, Inada Y, Nakano S, Tamura T, Takahashi T, Maruyama K, Yamazaki Y, Kuroda J, Shibata N: Effects of bezafibrate, PPARpan-agonist, and GW501516, PPARdelta agonist, on development of steatohepatitis in mice fed a methionine-and choline-deficient diet. Eur J Pharmacol 2006;536:182–191.
57 Oh KS, Kim M, Lee J, Kim MJ, Nam YS, Ham JE, Shin SS, Lee CM, Yoon M: Liver PPARalpha and UCP2 are involved in the regulation of obesity and lipid metabolism by swim training in genetically obese db/db mice. Biochem Biophys Res Commun 2006;345: 1232–1239.
58 Lee GY, Kim NH, Zhao ZS, Cha BS, Kim YS: Peroxisomal-proliferator-activated receptor alpha activates transcription of the rat hepatic malonyl-CoA decarboxylase gene: a key regulation of malonyl-CoA level. Biochem J 2004;378:983–990.
59 Minnich A, Tian N, Byan L, Bilder G: A potent PPARalpha agonist stimulates mitochondrial fatty acid beta-oxidation in liver and skeletal muscle. Am J Physiol Endocrinol Metab 2001;280:E270–E279.
60 Gilde AJ, Van Bilsen M: Peroxisome proliferator-activated receptors (PPARS): regulators of gene expression in heart and skeletal muscle. Acta Physiol Scand 2003;178:425–434.
61 Muoio DM, MacLean PS, Lang DB, Li S, Houmard JA, Way JM, Winegar DA, Corton JC, Dohm GL, Kraus WE: Fatty acid homeostasis and induction of lipid regulatory genes in skeletal muscles of peroxisome proliferator-activated receptor (PPAR) alpha knockout mice. Evidence for compensatory regulation by PPAR delta. J Biol Chem 2002;277: 26089–26097.
62 Wang YX, Lee CH, Tiep S, Yu RT, Ham J, Kang H, Evans RM: Peroxisome-proliferator-activated receptor delta activates fat metabolism to prevent obesity. Cell 2003;113: 159–170.
63 He J, Watkins S, Kelley DE: Skeletal muscle lipid content and oxidative enzyme activity in relation to muscle fiber type in type 2 diabetes and obesity. Diabetes 2001;50:817–823.
64 Wang YX, Zhang CL, Yu RT, Cho HK, Nelson MC, Bayuga-Ocampo CR, Ham J, Kang H, Evans RM: Regulation of muscle fiber type and running endurance by PPARdelta. PLoS Biol 2004;2:e294.
65 Abel ED, Peroni O, Kim JK, Kim YB, Boss O, Hadro E, Minnemann T, Shulman GI, Kahn BB: Adipose-selective targeting of the GLUT4 gene impairs insulin action in muscle and liver. Nature 2001;409:729–733,.
66 Knick B, Lange HJ, Heckmann K: Correlation between latent diabetes mellitus, obesity and fatty liver. Ger Med Mon 1966;11:149–152.
67 Lefebvre P, Chinetti G, Fruchart JC, Staels B: Sorting out the roles of PPAR alpha in energy metabolism and vascular homeostasis. J Clin Invest 2006;116:571–580.
68 Packard CJ: Triacylglycerol-rich lipoproteins and the generation of small, dense low-density lipoprotein. Biochem Soc Trans 2003;31:1066–1069.
69 Caslake MJ, Packard CJ, Gaw A, Murray E, Griffin BA, Vallance BD, Shepherd J: Fenofibrate and LDL metabolic heterogeneity in hypercholesterolemia. Arterioscler Thromb 1993;13:702–711.
70 Patsouris D, Mandard S, Voshol PJ, Escher P, Tan NS, Havekes LM, Koenig W, Marz W, Tafuri S, Wahli W, Muller M, Kersten S: PPARalpha governs glycerol metabolism. J Clin Invest 2004;114:94–103.
71 Tontonoz P, Hu E, Devine J, Beale EG, Spiegelman BM: PPAR gamma 2 regulates adipose expression of the phosphoenolpyruvate carboxykinase gene. Mol Cell Biol 1995;15: 351–357.
72 Devine JH, Eubank DW, Clouthier DE, Tontonoz P, Spiegelman BM, Hammer RE, Beale EG: Adipose expression of the phosphoenolpyruvate carboxykinase promoter requires peroxisome proliferator-activated receptor gamma and 9-cis-retinoic acid receptor binding to an adipocyte-specific enhancer in vivo. J Biol Chem 1999;274:13604–13612.
73 Holness MJ, Bulmer K, Smith ND, Sugden MC: Investigation of potential mechanisms regulating protein expression of hepatic pyruvate dehydrogenase kinase isoforms 2 and 4 by fatty acids and thyroid hormone. Biochem J 2003;369:687–695.
74 Page RL 2nd, Gozansky WS, Ruscin JM: Possible heart failure exacerbation associated with rosiglitazone: case report and literature review. Pharmacotherapy 2003;23:945–954.
75 Norris AW, Chen L, Fisher SJ, Szanto I, Ristow M, Jozsi AC, Hirshman MF, Rosen ED, Goodyear LJ, Gonzalez FJ, Spiegelman BM, Kahn CR: Muscle-specific PPARgamma-deficient mice develop increased adiposity and insulin resistance but respond to thiazolidinediones. J Clin Invest 2003;112:608–618.

76 Castrillo A, Tontonoz P: Nuclear receptors in macrophage biology: at the crossroads of lipid metabolism and inflammation. Annu Rev Cell Dev Biol 2004;20:455–480.

77 Babaev VR, Yancey PG, Ryzhov SV, Kon V, Breyer MD, Magnuson MA, Fazio S, Linton MF: Conditional knockout of macrophage PPARgamma increases atherosclerosis in C57BL/6 and low-density lipoprotein receptor-deficient mice. Arterioscler Thromb Vasc Biol 2005;25:1647–1653.

78 Selvaraj RK, Klasing KC: Lutein and eicosapentaenoic acid interact to modify iNOS mRNA levels through the PPARgamma/RXR pathway in chickens and HD11 cell lines. J Nutr 2006;136:1610–1616.

79 Klurfeld DM: Identification of foam cells in human atherosclerotic lesions as macrophages using monoclonal antibodies. Arch Pathol Lab Med 1985;109:445–449.

80 Pearson TA, Kramer EC, Solez K, Heptinstall RH: The human atherosclerotic plaque. Am J Pathol 1977;86:657–664.

81 Bouloumie A, Curat CA, Sengenes C, Lolmede K, Miranville A, Busse R: Role of macrophage tissue infiltration in metabolic diseases. Curr Opin Clin Nutr Metab Care 2005;8:347–354.

82 Welch JS, Ricote M, Akiyama TE, Gonzalez FJ, Glass CK: PPARgamma and PPARdelta negatively regulate specific subsets of lipopolysaccharide and IFN-gamma target genes in macrophages. Proc Natl Acad Sci USA 2003;100:6712–6717.

83 Pascual G, Fong AL, Ogawa S, Gamliel A, Li AC, Perissi V, Rose DW, Willson TM, Rosenfeld MG, Glass CK: A SUMOylation-dependent pathway mediates transrepression of inflammatory response genes by PPAR-gamma. Nature 2005;437:759–763.

84 Imbeault P, Lemieux S, Prud'homme D, Tremblay A, Nadeau A, Despres JP, Mauriege P: Relationship of visceral adipose tissue to metabolic risk factors for coronary heart disease: is there a contribution of subcutaneous fat cell hypertrophy? Metabolism 1999;48:355–362.

85 Szmitko PE, Wang CH, Weisel RD, de Almeida JR, Anderson TJ, Verma S: New markers of inflammation and endothelial cell activation: Part I. Circulation 2003;108:1917–1923.

86 Walczak R, Tontonoz P: PPARadigms and PPARadoxes: expanding roles for PPAR gamma in the control of lipid metabolism. J Lipid Res 2002;43:177–186.

87 Guo J, Van Eck M, de Waard V, Maeda N, Benson GM, Groot PH, Van Berkel TJ: The presence of leukocyte CC-chemokine receptor 2 in CCR2 knockout mice promotes atherogenesis. Biochim Biophys Acta 2005;1740:453–459.

88 Gu L, Okada Y, Clinton SK, Gerard C, Sukhova GK, Libby P, Rollins BJ: Absence of monocyte chemoattractant protein-1 reduces atherosclerosis in low density lipoprotein receptor-deficient mice. Mol Cell 1998;2:275–281.

89 Takahashi K, Takeya M, Sakashita N: Multifunctional roles of macrophages in the development and progression of atherosclerosis in humans and experimental animals. Med Electron Microsc 2002;35:179–203.

90 Li AC, Binder CJ, Gutierrez A, Brown KK, Plotkin CR, Pattison JW, Valledor AF, Davis RA, Willson TM, Witztum JL, Palinski W, Glass CK: Differential inhibition of macrophage foam-cell formation and atherosclerosis in mice by PPARalpha, beta/delta, and gamma. J Clin Invest 2004;114:1564–1576.

91 Febbraio M, Abumrad NA, Hajjar DP, Sharma K, Cheng W, Pearce SF, Silverstein RL: A null mutation in murine CD36 reveals an important role in fatty acid and lipoprotein metabolism. J Biol Chem 1999;274:19055–19062.

92 Chawla A, Boisvert WA, Lee CH, Laffitte BA, Barak Y, Joseph SB, Liao D, Nagy L, Edwards PA, Curtiss LK, Evans RM, Tontonoz P: A PPAR gamma-LXR-ABCA1 pathway in macrophages is involved in cholesterol efflux and atherogenesis. Mol Cell 2001;7:161–171.

93 Chinetti G, Lestavel S, Bocher V, Remaley AT, Neve B, Torra IP, Teissier E, Minnich A, Jaye M, Duverger N, Brewer HB, Fruchart JC, Clavey V, Staels B: PPAR-alpha and PPAR-gamma activators induce cholesterol removal from human macrophage foam cells through stimulation of the ABCA1 pathway. Nat Med 20017:53–58.

Journal of
Nutrigenetics
and
Nutrigenomics

J Nutrigenet Nutrigenomics 2008;1:136–151
DOI: 10.1159/000112461

Published online: February 20, 2008

Gene–Nutrient Interactions in the Metabolic Syndrome

Catherine M. Phillips Audrey C. Tierney Helen M. Roche

Nutrigenomics Research Group, Conway Institute, University College Dublin, Dublin, Ireland

Key Words
Metabolic syndrome · Dietary fatty acids · Gene–nutrient interaction · Insulin resistance · Obesity

Abstract
The metabolic syndrome (MetS) is a very common disease associated with an increased risk of type 2 diabetes mellitus and cardiovascular disease. The diverse clinical characteristics of the MetS illustrate the complexity of the disease process, which involves several dysregulated metabolic pathways. Thus, multiple genetic targets must be involved in the pathogenesis and progression of the disease. Research indicates a major role for genetic susceptibility to the MetS. However, the human genome has not changed markedly in the last decade but the prevalence of the condition has increased exponentially, illustrating the importance of gene–environmental interactions. Dietary fat is an important environmental factor which can modify the development of the MetS. Genetic background can interact with habitual dietary fat composition, affecting predisposition to the MetS. Recent research indicates that currently ineffective therapeutic dietary recommendations may require a 'personalised nutrition' approach, wherein the genetic profile may determine the responsiveness of patients to specific dietary fatty acid interventions. Understanding the biological impact of gene–nutrient interactions will provide a key insight into the pathogenesis and progression of diet-related polygenic disorders, including the MetS. This review will explore the interactions between genetic background and dietary exposure/nutritional therapy.

The Metabolic Syndrome – Definition, Prevalence and Preventative Strategies

The metabolic syndrome (MetS) is a very common, multi-component condition characterised by insulin resistance, dyslipidaemia, abdominal obesity and hypertension that is associated with an increased risk of type 2 diabetes mellitus (T2DM), cardiovascular disease (CVD) and atherosclerosis [1]. In 1970, Berson and Yallow [2] defined insulin resistance as 'a state (of a cell, tissue, system or body) in which greater-than-normal amounts of insulin are required to elicit a quantitatively normal response', resulting in an inability of insulin to provide normal glucose and lipid homeostasis. Reaven [3] hypothesised that insulin resistance, glucose intolerance and hyperinsulinaemia are the underlying components of the MetS or 'syndrome X', and increase the likelihood of other abnormalities occurring (dyslipidaemia, endothelial dysfunction, coagulation and inflammatory disorders and abnormal uric acid metabolism).

Insulin resistance is a key feature of obesity, the MetS, T2DM and CVD. The pathway that links obesity and insulin resistance with the MetS and T2DM represents a progressive phenotype (fig. 1) [4]. Surplus adipose tissue generates excessive metabolic stress (non-esterified fatty acids (NEFAs)) and pro-inflammatory adipocytokines (tumour necrosis factor-α, leptin, interleukin-6, angiotensinogen, plasminogen activator inhibitor type 1, etc.) that impede systemic responsiveness to insulin, resulting in impaired insulin action, compensatory hyperinsulinaemia and glucose intolerance [5–8]. Insulin resistance

KARGER

Fax +41 61 306 12 34
E-Mail karger@karger.ch
www.karger.com

1661–6499/08/0013–0136$24.50/0

Accessible online at:
www.karger.com/jnn

Helen M. Roche
Nutrigenomics Research Group, Conway Institute of Biomolecular and Biomedical Research, School of Public Health and Population Science
University College Dublin
Belfield, Dublin 4 (Ireland)
Tel. +353 1 716 6845, Fax +353 1 716 6701, E-Mail helen.roche@ucd.ie

leads to a variety of abnormalities in the liver, muscle and adipose tissue resulting in dyslipidaemia characterised by elevated NEFAs and triacylglycerol (TAG) concentrations and low high-density lipoprotein (HDL) levels. Individuals with a sensitive genotype and who are at increased risk of developing the MetS will be most susceptible to the impact of metabolic and pro-inflammatory stressors.

The World Health Organisation (WHO) criteria for defining the MetS focuses on risk for diabetes centred around impaired glucose tolerance (IGT), impaired fasting glucose or insulin resistance as measured by the hyperinsulinaemic euglycaemic clamp [9]. The International Diabetes Federation (IDF) definition focuses on central adiposity and the National Cholesterol Education Program (NCEP) Expert Panel on Detection, Evaluation, and Treatment of High Blood Cholesterol in Adults (Adult Treatment Panel (ATP) III) [10] assigns no priority to any of the criteria. In a recent perspective review, Reaven [11] summarised the similarities and differences of the three definitions of the MetS (WHO, IDF and ATPIII) but categorically stated that the components clustered in the syndrome occur only in insulin-resistant people. This is supported by results from animal studies [12, 13], and from human metabolic studies including the Insulin Resistance Atherosclerosis Study [14–16].

As there is no universal definition of the MetS, determination of the true global prevalence of the disease varies. Using the NCEP definition, the prevalence of the MetS is estimated to be 25% of the general population with no gender differences but varying with genetic background [17]. The IDF definition tends towards higher prevalence rates [18, 19]. Interestingly the WHO and the ATPIII of the NCEP definitions of the MetS have been shown to correlate closely in identifying people at risk of CVD [20]. Recently, Sandhofer et al. [21] compared the three definitions (WHO, IDF and ATPIII) with respect to metabolic parameters and their ability to predict intima media thickness and plaque extent in the carotid arteries. They found an increased prevalence of the MetS using the IDF criteria (25.8% for men and 19.5% for women). They also found that subjects identified by the WHO criteria (18.7% men; 16.2% women) had higher fasting insulin levels and were more insulin-resistant according to a higher homeostasis model assessment for insulin resistance than the subjects identified according to the NCEP ATPIII (18.9% men; 17.0% women) and the IDF criteria. They concluded that since the incidence of insulin resistance decreases with lower visceral obesity, using lower cut-off values decreases the specificity to detect insulin

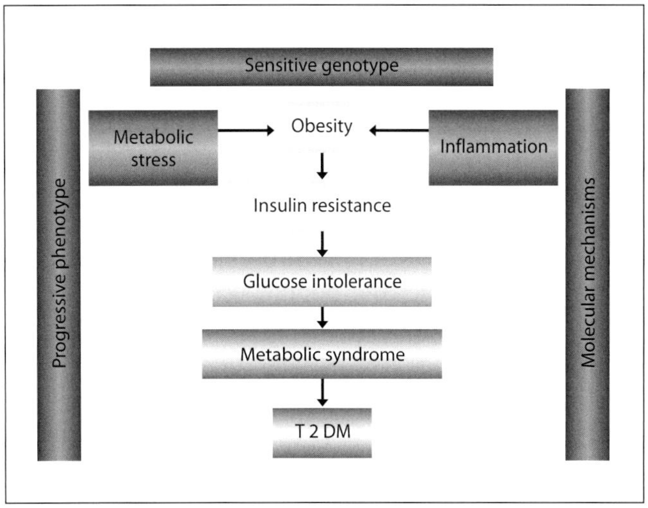

Fig. 1. The development and progression of the metabolic syndrome.

resistance [21]. Ford et al. [22] have reported an increase in the prevalence of the MetS from 23.1% in the National Health and Nutrition Examination Survey III (1988–1994) to 26.7% in the National Health and Nutrition Examination Survey (1999–2000).

Whilst diet and/or poor nutritional status are not risk factors for the MetS, reducing body weight, through manipulation of diet, is a well-accepted therapy to reduce the incidence of T2DM and improve risk factors such as hyperlipidaemia and hypertension. However poor compliance means that this therapeutic approach is largely ineffective and the prevalence of obesity continues to rise. Therefore other strategies to attenuate the impact of insulin resistance in the presence of obesity are required. Recently attention has shifted to the concept of 'personalised nutrition' wherein genetic testing preluding to appropriate nutritional or dietetic advice may be advocated. The exploration of genotype and diet and their interactions will be paramount both in new preventative programmes and in determining the risk of complex polygenic diet-related diseases [23], of which the MetS is at the forefront.

This article will review the evidence in relation to the genetic components of the MetS and then explore the hypothesis that this may be modified by dietary factors, in particular dietary fatty acid composition. Genetic background can determine an individual's responsiveness to altered dietary fatty acid composition, therefore dietary therapy to reduce the risk of the MetS may require a 'personalised' nutrition approach.

Genetic and Environmental Determinants of the Metabolic Syndrome

The current global epidemic in the incidence of the MetS and T2DM is an important illustration of the shared contribution of both genetic and environmental factors to diet-related polygenic disorders. Evidence for a genetic basis of the MetS and T2DM has been derived from studies of families, twins and populations with genetic admixture. The familial nature, the marked difference in the prevalence of the MetS among various racial groups and the difference in concordance rates between monozygotic twins are clearly consistent with a genetic component to disease susceptibility. High heritability estimates have been reported for fasting glucose, insulin, TAG and HDL cholesterol concentrations [24, 25]. Poulsen et al. [26] have studied the relative impact of genetic vs. environmental factors for the development of the components of the MetS amongst 303 elderly twin pairs. This study demonstrated that glucose intolerance, obesity and low HDL cholesterol concentrations are significantly higher among monozygotic twins than among dizygotic twins, indicating a genetic influence on the development on these phenotypes [26]. In contrast, the heritability estimates for hyperinsulinaemia, hypertension and hypertriacylglycerolaemia are low, indicating a more important environmental influence on these components of the MetS. More recently, results from a comprehensive study examining young and elderly monozygotic and dizygotic twins provided further evidence for a role of genes in controlling insulin secretion, insulin action and non-oxidative glucose metabolism [27]. These data indicate a major role for genetic susceptibility, whilst also emphasising the important role of the environment. In particular, trends in diet and physical activity, coupled with genetic susceptibility, must account for the recent and dramatic rise in the incidence of the MetS and T2DM, demonstrating the important impact of gene–environment interactions.

With the advent of high-throughput genetic analysis, our understanding of the genetic architecture and biology of diet-related polygenic disorders is improving. 2006 heralded identification of the most important T2DM susceptibility gene known so far, transcription factor 7-like 2 (TCF7L2) [28]. The original study in Icelandic, Danish and US white cohorts reported that single nucleotide polymorphisms (SNPs) of the TCF7L2 gene, especially rs12255372 and rs7903146, were strongly associated with T2DM [28]. This finding has been widely reproduced in several populations and also been shown to predict the conversion from IGT to overt diabetes [29]. More recently a Finnish study investigated the mechanisms of how these SNPs increase T2DM risk. They found that these variants altered TCF7L2 gene expression and are associated with decreased insulin secretion, but not insulin sensitivity, both in the general population as well as in T2DM offspring [30]. As part of this research the Finnish Diabetes Prevention Study investigated the association of these SNPs with incident diabetes. Five hundred and twenty-two overweight subjects with IGT were randomly assigned to either an intensive diet and lifestyle intervention group or a control group. Subjects in the intervention programme were given individually tailored dietary advice aimed to reduce weight and the intake of total and saturated fat and to increase the intake of dietary fibre. In addition, subjects were guided to increase their level of physical activity. The control group received general information on the benefits of weight reduction, physical activity and healthy diet. The mean duration of follow-up was 3.9 years, at which point DNA for genotyping was available from 507 subjects. Interestingly they found that variants were associated with incident diabetes in the control group, but not the intervention group. This indicates that environmental factors such as lifestyle intervention can reduce the risk conferred by genetic factors, even when risk genotypes are related to impaired insulin secretion [30].

There is no doubt that development of high-density arrays that permit the genotyping of hundreds of thousands of polymorphisms will rapidly advance our understanding of the genetic basis of T2DM, the MetS and obesity. A recent study [31] tested 392,935 SNPs in a French T2DM case-control cohort (n = 1,363). Markers with the most significant difference in genotype frequencies between T2DM cases and controls were fast-tracked for testing in a second cohort (n = 5,511). In addition to confirming the known association with the TCF7L2 gene, this study identified four loci containing variants that confer T2DM risk. These loci include a non-synonymous polymorphism in the zinc transporter SLC30A8, which is expressed exclusively in insulin-producing β-cells, and two linkage disequilibrium blocks that contain genes potentially involved in β-cell development or function (IDE-KIF11-HHEX and EXT2-ALX4). These associations may in part explain a substantial portion of disease risk and constitute proof of principle for the genome-wide approach to the elucidation of complex genetic traits [31]. Of the significantly associated SNPs in the French study, a number of these associations have been replicated in an Icelandic population in which 313,179 SNPs were tested for association with T2DM in a sample of 1,399

T2DM patients and 5,275 controls [32]. This study found that the TCF7L2 SNP rs7903146 conferred the most significant risk. In addition to confirming the association between the risk variants of SLC30A8 and HHEX with T2DM they also identified a variant in CDKAL1 that was associated with T2DM in European ancestry and Han Chinese ancestry. The insulin response for homozygotes was about 20% lower than for heterozygotes or non-carriers, indicating that this variant confers risk of T2DM through reduced insulin secretion. While the function of the gene product of CDKAL1 is unknown, the protein product is similar to another protein, CDK5 regulatory subunit-associated protein 1 (encoded by CDK5RAP1). In pancreatic β-cells CDK5 has been shown to play a role in the loss of β-cell function under glucotoxic conditions [33]. It is tempting to speculate that CDKAL1 may facilitate insulin production under such conditions through interaction with CDK5.

Genome-wide studies for T2DM susceptibility genes have also been useful in uncovering genes associated with obesity, a key feature of the MetS. Recently a common variant in the FTO gene that predisposes to diabetes through an effect on body mass index (BMI) has been identified [34]. This study compared 1,924 UK T2DM patients with 2,938 UK population controls for 490,032 autosomal SNPs. Polymorphisms in the FTO gene region on chromosome 16 were strongly associated with T2DM. They replicated this association in a further 3,757 T2DM cases and 5,346 controls. The 16% of adults who are homozygous for the risk allele weighed about 3 kg more and had a 1.67-fold increased risk of obesity when compared to those not carrying a risk allele. Furthermore the authors studied the association of FTO gene variation with BMI and the risk of being overweight and obese in an additional 19,424 white European adults and 10,172 white European children. These studies revealed that the T2DM-associated A allele of rs9939609 was associated with increased BMI and increased risk of being overweight and also being obese from childhood into old age [34]. While the function of the FTO gene is unknown, it lies adjacent to another gene, KIAA1005, which is transcribed in the opposite direction, opening up the possibility that genetic variation may affect a regulatory element for KIAA1005. Understanding the mechanisms whereby these variants influence the risk of obesity may provide insights into novel pathways involved in adiposity.

Prior to high-throughput large scale whole-genome-wide studies, genome scanning by positional cloning and the candidate gene approach have been the traditional techniques for identification of genes associated with T2DM and the MetS. Positional cloning involves mapping the susceptibility or causative loci purely on their chromosomal location using multi-generational pedigrees and/or a large number of sibling pairs. This approach allows identification of genes without any previous knowledge of biological function or the disease mechanism. However, to date this approach has identified relatively few candidate genes relevant to the MetS. The hepatic nuclear factor 4α (HNF4α) gene partly explains the linkage peak on chromosome 20 [35], while the upstream transcription factor (USF1) is associated with familial combined hyperlipidaemia and maps close to the T2DM-associated 1q peak [36–38]. Genome scanning in several different ethnic groups has identified chromosome regions harbouring T2DM susceptibility genes such as the novel gene, calpain 10 (CAPN10) [39]. Subsequent to this initial report, several groups have failed to show a relationship between CAPN10 and metabolic traits, or have shown modest associations for other sequence variations and/or haplotype combinations at the CAPN10 locus that might be associated with disease [40]. The lack of a consistent gene–phenotype relationship may be related to a number of causes of inconsistency in association studies, including population-specific patterns of linkage disequilibrium, population-specific environmental triggers, gene–gene interactions or gene–nutrient interactions.

The candidate gene approach identifies genes according to biological function and/or linkage studies, and association tests for significant differences in their allele frequencies between a patient group and a control population. Given the number of metabolic pathways involved in the MetS it is immediately apparent that the number of potential candidate genes is tremendous and overall, there has not been a high extent of success from candidate gene studies in terms of defining the genetic determinants of the MetS. Table 1 summarises the key pathways involved and some of the relevant candidate genes.

Monogenic forms of diabetes have identified several candidate genes for T2DM and the MetS. Six genes, glucokinase (GCK), insulin promoter factor-1 (IPF-1), neuro D1 transcription factor (NEUROD1), HNF-1β and HNF-4α, account for the majority of the 34 monogenic forms of diabetes [41]. Candidate gene association studies in T2DM indicate a role for a number of genes involved in insulin action as well as β-cell function [42, 43]. Fasting hyperglycaemia in T2DM is associated with a lack of inhibition of two key gluconeogenic enzymes, phosphoenolpyruvate carboxykinase (PEPCK) and glucose-6-

Table 1. Pathways adversely affected in the metabolic syndrome, and some of their relevant genes

Pathway	Genes involved
Insulin signalling	Forkhead box protein 1a (FOXO1A), glucose transporter 4 (SLC2A4), glycogen synthase kinase-3 (GSK3), insulin (INS), insulin promoter factor (IPF1), insulin receptor (INSR), insulin receptor substrates 1 and 2 (IRS1 and IRS2), phosphoinositide-3-kinase, regulatory subunit 1 (p85 α) (PIK3R1), phosphoinositide-3-kinase, regulatory subunit 2 (p85 β) (PIK3R2), protein kinase Bβ (AKT2), potassium channel inwardly rectifying subfamily J member 11 (KCNJ11), protein tyrosine phosphatase 1B (PTPN1), phosphatase and tensin homolog (PTEN), SH2-containing inositol phosphatase 2 (INPPL1), Son of sevenless homolog 1 (SOS1)
Glucose homeostasis	Calpain 10 (CAPN10), forkhead box O3A (FOXOA3), glucagon receptor (GCGR), glucokinase (GCK), glucose-6-phosphatase (G6PC), glucose transporters 2 and 4 (SLC2A2 and SLC2A4), glucose 6-phosphate transporter (SLC37A4), glycogen synthases 1 and 2 (GYS1 and GYS2), glycogen synthase kinases 3α and 3β (GSK3A and GSK3B) hexokinase 2 (HK2), hepatic nuclear factor 1α (TCF1), hepatic nuclear factor 1β (TCF2), hepatic nuclear factor 4α (HNF4A), phosphoenolpyruvate carboxykinase 1 (PCK1), upstream stimulatory factor 1 (USF1)
Lipoprotein metabolism	ATP-binding cassette, subfamily A, member 1 (ABCA1) ATP-binding cassette, subfamily G, member 5 (ABCG5), ATP-binding cassette, subfamily G, member 8 (ABCG8), apolipoproteins (APOA1, APOA2, APOA4, APOA5, APOB1, APOC2, APOC3, APOC4, APOE), acetoacyl-CoA thiolases 1 and 2 (ACAT1 and ACAT2), β_1- and β_2-adrenergic receptors (ADRB1 and ADRB2), CCAAT-enhancer-binding protein α (CEBPA), intestinal fatty acid-binding protein (FABP2), farnesoid X-activated receptor (NR1H4), liver X receptor α (NR1H3), lipoprotein lipase (LPL), peroxisome proliferator-activated receptors α, δ, and γ (PPARA, PPARD and PPARG), PPARγ co-activators 1α and 1β (PPARGC1A and PPARGC1B), retinoid X receptor α (RXRA), sterol regulatory element-binding proteins 1a and 1c (SREBF1a and SREBF1c), upstream stimulatory factor 1 (USF1), VLDL receptor (VLDLR)
Adipogenesis and inflammation	Adipocyte fatty acid-binding protein (FABP4), adiponectin (ADIPOQ), CCAAT-enhancer-binding proteins α and β (CEBPA and CEBPβ), ghrelin (GHRL), interleukin 6 (IL6), leptin (LEP), leptin receptor (LEPR), resistin (RETN), tumour necrosis factor α (TNF), uncoupling proteins 1, 2 and 3 (UCP1, UCP2 and UCP3)
Vascular function and coagulation	Angiotensinogen (AGT), angiotensin-converting enzyme (ACE), β_1- and β_2-adrenergic receptors (ADRB1 and ADRB2), endothelial nitric oxide synthase (NOS3), fibrinogen α and β polypeptides (FGA and FGB), inducible nitric oxide synthase (NOS2A), plasminogen activator inhibitor type 1 (SERPINE1), tissue plasminogen activator (PLAT), endothelin-1 (EDN1), von Willebrand factor (VWF)

phosphatase (G6Pase) which are regulated at the transcriptional level by insulin through protein kinase B (PKB) [44]. The essential role of PKBβ (or AKT2) in insulin signalling and maintenance of glucose homeostasis was demonstrated by the finding of a missense mutation in AKT2 in a family with severe insulin resistance and diabetes [45]. PKB also regulates the peroxisome proliferator-activated receptor γ (PPARγ) coactivator (PGC1) [46], the transcriptional co-activator which interacts with HNF4α, PPARγ and forkhead transcription factor 1 (Foxo1) to execute hepatic gluconeogenesis. Impaired insulin signalling and glucose metabolism within the context of insulin resistance have been comprehensively reviewed elsewhere [47]. This review will focus on recent advances of well-characterised, common genetic variants of lipid-related genes associated with the MetS.

Dyslipidaemia is one of the very early features of the MetS and frequently precedes IGT. A number of lipid-sensitive transcription factors, including FXR, LXRα, RXRα, PPARα, PPARδ, PGC1α, PGC1β, SREBP-1a and SREBP-1c, have been implicated in the development of the MetS. PPARγ is a good candidate gene for the MetS because of its multiple roles in adipocyte differentiation, fatty acid metabolism, insulin sensitivity and glucose homeostasis [48–50]. Up until recently the Pro12Ala PPARγ polymorphism had been identified as the most widely reproduced genetic variation for the risk of T2DM [40]. The original study investigating the polymorphism in T2DM demonstrated that the alanine allele of the Pro12Ala PPARγ polymorphism was associated with lower BMI, improved insulin sensitivity and thus reduced diabetes risk by 75% [51]. However not all associations with this polymorphism were consistent [52–55] and those reports that have confirmed the association [56] have shown that the apparent protective effect of the PPARγ polymorphism is to a much lesser extent. Thus, a large association study of 3,000 subjects supported by a meta-analysis of 16 previously published studies has been conducted to overcome the inherent limitations of the smaller individual studies [57]. This study confirmed a modest (1.25-fold) but significant increase in diabetes risk for the Pro12Pro genotype [57]. More recently the contribution of the Pro12 allele to the genetic risk of T2DM was confirmed in a French Caucasian population, the Pro12 allele almost doubled risk particularly in obese subjects. Interestingly the obese phenotype seemed to exacerbate the detrimental effect of the PPARγ Pro12 allele on insulin sensitivity [58]. The Pro12Pro genotype also predicts the conversion from IGT to T2DM, Pro12 homozygotes had a 2.9-fold greater risk of developing diabetes compared to Ala12 carriers [59]. Haplotype studies have demonstrated that the Ala12 variant of PPARγ modulates susceptibility to T2DM in concert with other variants at the PPARγ locus. Doney et al. [60] showed that the Ala12 variant conferred protection in haplotypes not containing the 1431T variant, but the presence of 1431T in the haplotype (70% of Ala12 carriers) abolished protection. Interestingly, another recent study of four common PPARγ polymorphisms (–681C/T, –689C/T, Pro12Ala, and 1431C/T) found no impact of individual polymorphisms on the MetS. However haplotype analyses revealed a significant enrichment of the GTGC haplotype frequency (constituted by the –681C/T, –689C/T, Pro12Ala, and 1431C/T polymorphisms in this order) among subjects with the MetS [61]. These data support the suggestion that PPARγ gene variation may increase the risk of the MetS.

Disturbed lipoprotein metabolism is a key feature of the MetS, characterised by elevated TAG and low HDL cholesterol concentrations. One of the new potential candidate genes is the scavenger receptor class B type I (SR-BI or SCARB1) gene. SCARB1, a cell-surface glycoprotein, was the first HDL receptor to be defined and characterised. Acton et al. [62] described three common variants (at exon 1 [G/A], exon 8 [C/T], and intron 5 [C/T]), which were associated with HDL cholesterol, triglycerides, and BMI, suggesting that SCARB1 might be involved in determining some features of the MetS. In terms of the relations between HDL and triglyceride-rich lipoproteins (TRLs), the lipase gene family (hepatic lipase (LIPC), lipoprotein lipase (LPL), endothelial lipase (LIPG), and pancreatic lipase (PL)) represents a growing and promising superfamily in which common variations have been related to HDL cholesterol and TAG metabolism, but also sporadically with blood pressure, obesity, and insulin resistance. Numerous variants within the LPL gene, which hydrolyses core TAG from circulating TRLs that are then either degraded by the liver or converted to LDL particles by LIPG, have been identified (i.e., *Hin*dIII, S447X, D9N, and N291S), and they have been widely associated with HDL cholesterol and TAG concentrations [63]. However, some differences among studies and populations suggest the presence of interactions with additional factors [63]. A recent study examined the associations of LIPG haplotypes with lipoprotein risk factors in 541 adult Japanese Americans and found stronger associations for HDL_3 cholesterol and plasma apolipoprotein AI levels [64]. Numerous polymorphisms have also been analyzed in the hepatic lipase gene. Four SNPs in the promoter region (–250G/A, –514C/T, –710T/C, and –763A/G) are in strong linkage disequilibrium, and they have been associated with HDL cholesterol and TAG levels, with important differences among studies depending on the ethnic, anthropometric, and dietary characteristics of the populations [65].

Finally, several variants of the APOA1/C3/A4/A5 and APOE/C1/C2 gene clusters have been consistently associated with the characteristic dyslipidaemia of the MetS [66]. Lai et al. [67] have investigated five polymorphisms of the newly identified ApoAV gene, which lies close to the APOAI/CIII/AIV gene cluster, in several Asian populations and in the Framingham population, which is mostly of European descent. In all populations, the –1131T/C polymorphism had an important impact on plasma TAG and HDL cholesterol. In addition, the rare alleles of the –1464T/C, –1131T/C, S19W, and 1259T/C SNPs were each significantly associated with elevated TAG levels (19–86 mg/dl) and had clear gene-dose effects [68]. The Ala54Thr polymorphism in the fatty acid-binding protein 2 (FABP2) gene as well as the –455T/C and –482C/T polymorphisms in the apolipoprotein C-III (APOC3) gene promoter have been associated with features of the MetS in specific populations [69]. Guettier et al. [69] evaluated the association between these polymorphisms in Asian-Indians with the MetS and dyslipidaemia. Controls carrying FABP2 Thr54 were more likely to have the MetS than non-carriers. Those carrying at least one polymorphic allele in both genes had a higher likelihood of having the MetS and dyslipidaemia than wild-type [69].

In conclusion these data indicate a major role for genetic susceptibility to the MetS. However, regardless of the approach used, genetic disease-association studies are fraught with difficulties, and a number of the positive results have not been replicated in subsequent studies [70]. The main reasons for the disparity are inadequate statistical power, multiple hypothesis testing, population stratification, publication bias and phenotypic differences. It is becoming increasingly evident that the identification of true genetic associations in common multi-factorial conditions, such as the MetS, requires large studies consisting of thousands rather than hundreds of subjects. Also, the absence of large single-gene effects and the detection of multiple small effects accentuate the need for the study of larger populations in order to reliably identify the size of the effect now expected for complex diseases. The discovery of associated variants in unsuspected genes and outside coding regions illustrates the ability of genome-wide association studies to provide potentially important clues into the pathogenesis of common diseases. However it is also important to bear in mind that the human genome has not significantly changed in the last decade but the prevalence of the MetS has increased exponentially, illustrating the importance of gene–environment interactions.

Nutrient Determinants of the Metabolic Syndrome – Dietary Fat Composition

In addition to elevated fasting glucose concentrations, the insulin-resistant subject displays an imbalance in fatty acid metabolism reflected by increased levels of circulating NEFAs and TAG. This metabolic phenotype is exacerbated in the obese state [71] and inhibits insulin-stimulated glucose uptake into muscle. In this insulin-resistant state, NEFA levels are increased both in the fasted and the fed state [72]. In obesity, adipose tissue is resistant to the anti-lipolytic effect of insulin, and becomes limited in its ability to store lipids. Consequently, an increase in circulating NEFAs occurs leading to an imbalance between the oxidation of fat and of glucose [73]. It has been proposed that abnormal accumulation of fat in muscle and other tissues leads to lipotoxicity, induced β-cell failure, hyperglycaemia, increased plasma NEFA concentrations and increased VLDL production, all playing an important role in the aetiology of insulin resistance [74].

NEFAs have an important stimulatory effect on glucose-stimulated insulin secretion (GSIS) by maintaining a basal rate of insulin secretion and in turn regulating adipose tissue lipolysis. In the MetS and T2DM, increased NEFAs contribute to hyperinsulinaemia and ultimately overexposure results in β-cell damage. It has been proposed that elevation in the basal glucose level increases glucose-derived malonyl-CoA within the β-cell [75]. Increased levels of intracellular malonyl-CoA inhibit the activity of carnitine palmitoyl transferase-1 (CPT-1) resulting in increased long-chain acyl-CoA levels [76]. The malonyl-CoA–CPT-1 interaction is central to GSIS, highlighting the role of fatty acids in the process [74]. The insulinotrophic effects of NEFAs differ with respect to the level of saturation. In one study, endogenous circulating NEFAs were eliminated with the anti-lipolytic agent nicotinic acid and replaced with soybean oil (which is predominantly polyunsaturated fatty acids (PUFAs)) or lard oil (a source of saturated fatty acids (SFAs)). After a glucose challenge, the proportion of insulin secretion was far more effective after the SFA treatment [77]. This study also demonstrated that GSIS increased dramatically with chain length and degree of unsaturation (C8:0, C18:2, C18:1, C16:0, C18:0). Other animal studies have displayed a potent effect of increased islet TAG content on β-cell function [78]. This fat accumulation in the islets and its subsequent effects on GSIS warrants further investigation.

Disruption of the insulin-signalling cascade by increased NEFA- or fatty acid-derived products including TAG has a negative impact on insulin sensitivity. These effects are well characterised in muscle [79]. The insulin-signalling cascade involves a sequence of reactions in which binding of insulin to the insulin receptor (IR) causes tyrosine phosphorylation of insulin receptor substrate-1 (IRS-1). Subsequent activation of phosphatidylinositol (PI) 3-kinase facilitates translocation of glucose transporter 4 (GLUT4) to the plasma membrane resulting in increased glucose transport into the cells [80]. Circulating NEFAs (malonyl-CoA, long-chain acyl-CoA) reduce muscle glucose oxidation and glycogen synthesis by impairing glucose transport [81] and impeding insulin-mediated tyrosine phosphorylation of IRS-1 and IRS-1-associated PI3 kinase activity, which is associated with a substantial increase in membrane-bound protein kinase C theta (PKCθ), a known serine kinase. LC-acyl-CoA generates a pool of diacylglycerol which may activate PKCθ. Phosphorylation of IRS-1 on a serine residue affects GLUT4 translocation to the cell surface [74]. A similar mechanism involving IRS-2 is suggested to occur in the liver [80]. As the IR is a membrane-bound protein and its function is membrane-dependent, it is reasonable to speculate that a change in membrane lipid induced by dietary fat may impact on the function of the plasma membrane IR [81]. In isolated rat adipocytes, it has been demonstrated that a high PUFA:SFA diet increased IR function, glucose oxidation and glucose transport [82]. A high-PUFA diet can also increase receptor tyrosine kinase activity [83]. Again these dietary effects may be further modulated by the degree of unsaturation and chain length of the unsaturated fatty acids.

There is increasing evidence that the composition of the diet, in terms of quality and quantity of fat, plays an important role in glucose homeostasis and insulin sensitivity. It is generally agreed that saturated fats have a detrimental effect on lipoproteins and on insulin sensitivity whilst unsaturated fats have a more beneficial outcome. Animal and human studies have demonstrated that SFAs increase insulin resistance [84–87]. Studies determining the effect of monounsaturated fatty acids (MUFAs) on insulin resistance have demonstrated improved peripheral insulin sensitivity following MUFA-rich diets in both healthy [88, 89] and diabetic cohorts [90]. However, the effect of MUFAs on insulin resistance is still somewhat controversial since it has been suggested that dietary oleic acid influences fat oxidation [91], which may in turn have a negative effect on insulin sensitivity. The role of n–6 and n–3 PUFAs on insulin sensitivity remains controversial [6, 92].

While there is clear evidence from epidemiological and cohort studies of the detrimental effects of total fat (particularly SFA) on insulin resistance and the development of T2DM [93–96], the optimal amount and type of dietary fat for the prevention of insulin resistance and the MetS remains unclear. Diets rich in MUFAs tend to improve insulin sensitivity [97, 98], however not all studies have shown a positive effect [91, 99]. A number of studies have also focused on the relative effect of substituting SFA with MUFA or carbohydrate, since high-carbohydrate diets have been associated with increased TAG concentrations, reduced HDL cholesterol concentrations [90, 100] and reduced glycaemic control.

The anti-atherogenic effects of PUFAs are well documented [101]. However their effects on insulin sensitivity are less well defined. In vitro and animal studies have shown encouraging effects of PUFAs on insulin action [102], especially with fish oils of which long-chain n–3 PUFAs such as eicosapentaenoic acid (EPA) and docosahexaenoic acid (DHA) are found in high concentrations [103]. Laaksonen et al. [104] showed an association of the n–6 PUFA linoleate in serum with the risk of development of impaired fasting glucose or diabetes in middle-aged men over a 4-year follow-up. Salmeron et al. [105] postulated a reduction in T2DM by replacing 2% of energy from *trans* fatty acids isoenergetically with PUFAs, indicating that increased intakes of long-chain PUFAs reduce insulin resistance. Animal studies have confirmed this, showing significant decreases in lipids, glucose levels and an increase in insulin sensitivity [106]. Intake of fish oils directly influences the fatty acid composition of membrane phospholipids [103] and increases insulin sensitivity [107, 108]. n–3 PUFAs require sufficient duration to effect a compositional change in cell membrane phospholipids in order for their direct action on insulin resistance to be assessed, in contrast to their established indirect effect on endothelial function, platelet aggregation, TAG concentration and arrhythmic effects [109]. Animal studies have shown that a diet rich in long-chain n–3 PUFAs (EPA and DHA) prevented insulin resistance in muscle and liver, through the hypothesised effect of reducing fat content in muscle and thus maintaining normal PI3 kinase activity and expression and translocation of GLUT4 receptors and by inhibiting hepatic glucose production in the liver [84].

In contrast there is limited and conflicting epidemiological data regarding the effects of fish and fish oil supplements in humans on insulin sensitivity. The Seven Countries Study [110] and the Nurses Health Study [105] showed inverse associations between fish consumption and glucose concentrations and the incidence of T2DM. However other studies have failed to replicate these findings [111]. In the KANWU study, supplementation with n–3 PUFAs did not influence insulin sensitivity on the high-fat or high-MUFA diets, confirming the controversial effects of n–3 PUFAs in human interventions as opposed to animal models.

Numerous intervention studies determining the effect of total fat intake on insulin sensitivity (measured by the clamp technique or variations in the frequently sampled intravenous glucose tolerance test) have shown that high-fat diets (>38% energy from fat) exacerbate insulin resistance. Low-fat diets, however, have been shown to have a beneficial effect [99, 112–114]. Categorising people by BMI was shown to increase insulin sensitivity in the more overweight and obese categories when total dietary fat is reduced [91]. The use of 24-hour recalls and weighed food diaries in estimating diet composition are adequate but not ideal. Underreporting of dietary fat, carbohydrate, and frequency of snacking and over-emphasis of a healthy eating type pattern is repeatedly observed in dietary studies, especially in overweight and obese recorders. As a complementary and more reliable or valid marker of habitual diet, fatty acid composition of serum lipid esters can be measured. Vessby [115] found higher proportions of SFAs in T2DM patients compared with healthy controls. Vessby et al. [116] subsequently measured the fatty acid composition of serum cholesterol esters, representative of the dietary fat composition for the previous 6–8 weeks, in 70-year-old men. Insulin sensitivity was associated with low proportions of palmitic (C16:0) and palmitoleic (C16:1n–7) acids and a high proportion of linoleic acid (C18:2n–6) [116]. The fatty acid profiles of the insulin-resistant subjects suggest possible changes in the activities of desaturation (↓Δ5-desaturase, ↑Δ6- and Δ9-desaturase) and elongation enzymes [115] indicating that these enzymes are insulin-dependent. These desaturase activity profiles have also been observed with obesity and lifestyle factors in men and women [117]. Clearly disturbed fatty acid metabolism, which may be secondary to excessive/imbalanced dietary fat intake, may be involved in the pathogenesis of the MetS. More recently, Warensjo et al. [118] identified specific fatty acid factors as measures of dietary fat quality and endogenous fatty acid metabolism in relation to the MetS. Using principal factor analysis on fatty acid profiles of men participating in a population-based cohort study, the Uppsala Longitudinal Study of Adult Men, factors were generated at ages 50 (n = 2,009) and 70 (n = 576) years, and relations between fatty acid factors and the MetS (National Cholesterol Education Program) were studied in cross-sectional and prospective (20 years) analyses. They identified 3 major fatty acid factors: a low-linoleic acid factor, a dietary saturated fatty acid factor, and an n–3 polyunsaturated fatty acid factor. All factors differed between those subjects with the MetS (n = 281 of 2,009) and those without the MetS at age 50 years; only the low-linoleic acid factor differed at age 70 years, suggesting an association between the MetS and fat quality. The low-linoleic acid factor and the n–3 PUFA factor predicted the development of the MetS over 20 years, independent of smoking habits, physical activity, and BMI. This finding supports current dietary recommendations to increase PUFA and restrict SFA intakes.

Gene–Nutrient Interactions: Implications for Dietary Fatty Acids

In light of the Human Genome Project and the rapid advances in molecular biology, a wealth of genetic information is being generated, particularly with respect to the common, polygenic, diet-related diseases including obesity, insulin resistance, the MetS and T2DM. It is becoming increasingly obvious that an individual's phenotype represents a complex interaction between the genetic background and environmental factors over the course of an individual's lifetime. Food intake and nutrient exposure are key environmental factors in the pathogenesis and progression of the common polygenic, diet-related diseases. Therefore it is time to identify the nutrient-sensitive genotypes and to develop a 'personalised nutrition' approach, whereby nutrient intake is manipulated/optimised based on an individual's genetic profile to reduce disease risk and/or improve the effectiveness of dietary guidelines/recommendations.

It is well known that the effect of dietary changes on plasma biomarker concentrations differs significantly between individuals. Currently, there is considerable support for the notion that the inter-individual variability in response to dietary modification is determined by genetic factors – this is especially true for lipid and lipoprotein phenotypes [119]. Insulin resistance precedes the development of MetS and T2DM. Genes and the environment determine insulin resistance. The 'thrifty genotype' [120], arising from evolutionary selection of genes that were originally beneficial for energy storage and which conferred a protective effect in times of food deprivation by promoting fat deposition, has been proposed to explain the current escalating incidence of obesity in a modern environment of physical inactivity and excessive energy intake. This review will explore the interactions between genetic background and an individual's nutrient exposure, with particular focus on dietary fatty acid composition.

As previously mentioned hepatic lipase (HL) is a lipolytic enzyme that plays a role in the metabolism of several lipoproteins, while insulin up-regulates the activity of HL via insulin-responsive elements in the HL promoter. Results from the Hoorn Study suggest that higher intakes of total and saturated fat were positively associated with higher HL activity. Furthermore they reported that the observed association between total fat and HL activity was modified by the –514C/T polymorphism of the hepatic lipase gene, with stronger associations observed between total dietary fat intake and HL activity in subjects with the CT and TT genotypes compared to CC homozygotes [121]. Data from NUGENOB, a study investigating genotype-by-nutrient interactions in obesity, in which 42 polymorphisms of 26 candidate genes for obesity were genotyped in 549 adult obese women recruited from eight European centres in a case-only study, reported an interaction between the –514C/T HL gene polymorphism and fibre intake. They also found interactions between the –11377G/C polymorphism of the adiponectin gene (ADIPOQ) and the –681C/G polymorphism of the PPARG3 gene, with the percentage of energy derived from fat in the diet for the development of obesity. However it must be noted that this study was case-only in design and did not take multiple testing into account, therefore these results should be considered with caution [122]. Ordovas et al. [123] investigated the interaction effects between the –514C/T polymorphism, dietary fat and HDL-related measures in 1,020 men and 1,110 women participating in the Framingham Study. They found that the T allele was only associated with higher HDL cholesterol levels and size in subjects consuming <30% of energy from fat. When total fat was ≥30% of energy mean HDL cholesterol levels were lowest in the TT homozygotes and no difference was observed in the CT and CC individuals. These correlations were observed for SFA and MUFA (particularly for animal fat), but not for PUFA. One interpretation of these results could be that in the Framingham Study, TT subjects may have an impaired adaptation to higher animal fat diets and could result in higher cardiovascular risk.

Gene–diet interactions between the APOA5 gene variation and PUFAs in relation to plasma lipid concentrations and lipoprotein particle size have been reported [124]. Furthermore, it has been shown that obesity modulates the effect of the APOA5 gene variation in carotid intima media thickness, a surrogate measure of atherosclerosis [125]. More recently the same group reported that the –1131T/C polymorphism in the APOA5 gene modulates the effect of fat intake on BMI and obesity risk in both men and women in the Framingham Study [126]. The interaction with BMI was dose-dependent, and no statistically significant heterogeneity by gender was detected. In subjects homozygous for the –1131T major allele, BMI increased as total fat intake increased. Conversely, this increase was not present in carriers of the –1131C minor allele. When specific fatty acid groups were analyzed, MUFAs showed the highest statistical significance for these interactions with obesity-related measures (BMI, overweight, and obesity).

Apolipoprotein CIII (apo CIII) is a marker of CVD risk associated with TAG-rich lipoproteins. The –455T/C polymorphism in the insulin-responsive element of the apo CIII gene influences TAG and apo CIII concentrations. A formal interactive effect between apo CIII genotype and n–3 PUFAs was confirmed by logistic models in the study of Oliveri et al. [127]. Patients homozygous for the –455C apo CIII variant are poorly responsive to the apo C-III-lowering effects of n–3 PUFAs [127].

Apolipoprotein E is a structural component of several lipoproteins, and serves as a ligand for the LDL receptor and the LDL receptor-related protein. The *APOE* gene promoter –219G/T polymorphism is associated with coronary heart disease and increased postprandial TRL levels [128], and susceptibility of LDL to oxidative modifications [129], circumstances related to insulin resistance. The effect of this polymorphism on peripheral insulin sensitivity was investigated using the insulin suppression test after the consumption of three diets: high MUFA, high SFA and high carbohydrate. The steady-state plasma glucose concentration was lower in GG subjects than in GT and TT individuals, regardless of the diet consumed. Significant diet–genotype interactions were found for steady-state plasma glucose and NEFA concentrations. Thus the shift from the SFA-rich diet to the MUFA- or carbohydrate-rich diets decreased the steady-state plasma glucose and NEFA concentrations in GG and GT subjects, but not in TT subjects [130].

Scavenger receptor class B type I (SCARB1) mediates the absorption of dietary cholesterol in the intestine, suggesting that it may also play a role in postprandial responses. The presence of the 2 allele at the SR-BI polymorphism in exon 1 was associated with faster clearance of small TRLs, probably due to a more rapid hepatic uptake [131]. Increasing evidence indicates that SCARB1 plays additional roles particularly in T2DM. More recently, it has been reported that carriers of the G/A genotype have significant increases in insulin sensitivity after a MUFA-rich diet compared with G/G individuals [132].

The intestinal fatty acid-binding protein (IFBP), coded by the FABP2 gene, is one of the most abundant proteins in enterocytes and genetic variation at this locus was associated with insulin resistance in Pima Indians. In particular the Ala54Thr polymorphism has been associated with hypertriglyceridaemia and insulin resistance. Marin et al. [133] showed that insulin sensitivity decreased in subjects with the Thr54 allele when SFAs were replaced by MUFAs and carbohydrates. However, no significant differences between the 3 diets were observed in the Ala54 allele homozygotes.

PPARs are members of the nuclear-hormone receptor superfamily of which there are three isoforms PPARα, PPARβ/δ and PPARγ. Unsaturated fatty acids can bind to specific isoforms and activate PPARs. This binding varies according to the PPAR's affinity which is dependent on fatty acid chain length and degree of unsaturation. Recent studies have suggested that n–3 fatty acids protect against high-fat diet-induced insulin resistance through PPAR activation and a subsequent decrease in intracellular lipid abundance [134]. Tai et al. [135] have shown that the Leu162Val polymorphism of the PPARα gene effects plasma TG and apoC-III concentrations depending on the dietary PUFA, with a high intake triggering lower TG in carriers of the 162V allele. Furthermore, the PPARα Leu162Val polymorphism may contribute to inter-individual variability in plasma lipoprotein and lipid response after modification of the dietary PUFA:SFA ratio [136].

It has been demonstrated that several n–3 and n–6 PUFAs activate PPARγ [137]. In the context of insulin resistance, PPARγ regulates adipogenesis and is involved in insulin sensitisation [137]. PPARγ promotes the storage of fat and increases adipocyte differentiation and enhances the transcription of genes important for lipogenesis [138]. The PPARγ Pro12Ala polymorphism provides an excellent example of the relevance of gene–nutrient interactions in the development of the MetS and T2DM. In a prospective population-based cohort study, Luan et al. [139] demonstrated an important interaction between habitual dietary fat composition and the PPARγ Pro12Ala polymorphism. They found that as the PUFA:SFA ratio increased a significant inverse relationship was shown for both fasting insulin concentrations and BMI in the Ala carriers, suggesting that the potential protective effect of the Ala allele may be lost in the presence of a high SFA diet. The Quebec Family Study [140] has also demonstrated that the PPARγ Pro12Ala polymorphism modulates the relationship between dietary fat intake and components of the MetS. In this study it was found that total fatty acid and SFA intakes are correlated with BMI, visceral adipose tissue area, waist circumference and fasting glucose concentrations in Pro12 homozygotes, but these associations are not observed among carriers of the Ala allele. Also, when the two genotype groups are classified according to quartiles of total fatty acid and SFA intakes, the positive correlation between fat and waist circumference remains in the Pro12 homozygotes, but again there is no relationship in the Ala carriers [140]. Thus, there is a disparity between the results of these two studies that have investigated the interaction between the PPARγ Pro12Ala polymorphism and dietary fatty acids. While the discrepancies may be population-specific, both studies highlight the need to take account of diet-related environmental exposure and the relevance of gene–nutrient interactions, particularly in relation to the possible role of dietary fatty acids in the MetS. More recently, a direct relationship between the intake of *trans* fatty acids and T2DM in the Ala carriers of the polymorphism has been reported [141]. The authors speculate that from a biological point of view it is plausible for *trans* fatty acids to have the same effect as saturated fatty acids in activation of the steatosis pathways that result in insulin resistance and early β-cell dysfunction.

It is worth noting that while other studies have also reported this gene–nutrient interaction [140] the results have not been consistent with the original findings of Luan et al. [139], and others have failed to show a gene–nutrient interaction between the PPARγ polymorphism and dietary fatty acid composition [142]. One study also reported that the Ala12 allele was associated with an increased risk of progression to T2DM, however the Ala12Ala genotype was associated with increased weight loss in response to lifestyle intervention and less progression from IGT to T2DM [143]. More recently Scacchi et al. [144] analysed the distribution of this polymorphism and prevalence of T2DM in world populations in relation to dietary habits. In European populations the Ala allele frequencies are distributed according to a latitudinal trend, with the highest in northern and central European populations and the lowest in the Mediterranean populations. An inverse relationship between Ala frequency and T2DM prevalence was observed mainly in populations where energy from lipids exceeded 30% of the total energy intake. While the focus of this review is on environmental factors, in particular dietary fat, it should be noted that non-environmental factors should also be considered and recent studies have shown that physical activity interacts with the PPARγ Pro12Ala polymorphism and has effects on fasting insulin concentrations, a surrogate marker for insulin resistance [145, 146].

Conclusions

The recent global epidemic of the MetS is an important illustration of how nutrient exposure and genetic background can dramatically impact on the development of the disease. Clearly, there is ample evidence to suggest that an individual's genetic background can interact with their dietary fat exposure to affect risk of the MetS. To date, most studies have focused on a limited number of genetic variants. More comprehensive genetic/nutrient analysis in larger cohorts is needed to confirm these findings. Nevertheless, the preliminary data provide an interesting concept worthy of further study, in terms of both gene–nutrient interactions modulating the risk of onset of the MetS and therapeutic dietary interventions. Indeed, in the future a 'personalised nutrition' approach may be advocated, wherein patients with a particular genetic profile(s) may determine responsiveness to specific dietary fatty acid interventions. With the advent of high-throughput genetic analysis our understanding of the genetic basis of diet-related polygenic disorders should improve, allowing the implementation of more effective patient risk assessment and personalised nutritional therapies. Only with a full understanding of multiple gene–gene, gene–nutrient and gene–nutrient–environment interactions can the molecular basis of the MetS be solved in order to reduce the risk and minimise the adverse health effects of obesity, T2DM and CVD.

Disclosure Statement

The authors declare that no financial or other conflict of interest exists in relation to the content of the article.

References

1 Moller DE, Kaufman KD: Metabolic syndrome: a clinical and metabolic perspective. Annu Rev Med 2004;56:45–62.

2 Berson SA, Yallow RS: Insulin 'antagonists' and insulin resistance; in Ellenberg M, Rifkin H (eds): Diabetes Mellitus: Theory and Practice New York, McGraw Hill, 1970, pp 388–423.

3 Reaven G: Banting Lecture 1988. Role of insulin resistance in human disease. Diabetes 1988;37:1595–1607.

4 Roche HM: Fatty acids and the metabolic syndrome. Proc Nutr Soc 2005;64:23–29.

5 Schinner S, Scherbaum WA, Bornstein WA, Barthel A: Molecular mechanisms of insulin resistance. Diabet Med 2005;22:674–682.

6 Roche HM, Phillips C, Gibney MJ: The metabolic syndrome: the crossroads of diet and genetics. Proc Nutr Soc 2005;64:371–377.

7 Ghanim H, Aljada A, Hofmeyer D, Syed T, Mohanty P, Dandona P: Circulating mononuclear cells in the obese are in a proinflammatory state. Circulation 2004;110:1564–1571.

8 Saltiel AR: The molecular and physiological basis of insulin resistance: emerging implications for metabolic and cardiovascular diseases. J Clin Invest 2000;106:163–164.

9 Alberti KG, Zimmet PZ: Definition, diagnosis and classification of diabetes mellitus and its complications. Part 1: diagnosis and classification of diabetes mellitus provisional report of a WHO consultation. Diabet Med 1998;15:539–553.

10 Expert Panel on Detection, Evaluation, and Treatment of High Blood Cholesterol in Adults: Executive Summary of The Third Report of The National Cholesterol Education Program (NCEP) Expert Panel on Detection, Evaluation, And Treatment of High Blood Cholesterol In Adults (Adult Treatment Panel III). JAMA 2001;285:2486–2497.

11 Reaven GM: The metabolic syndrome: is this diagnosis necessary? Am J Clin Nutr 2006; 83:1237–1247.

12 Shafrir E: Development and consequences of insulin resistance: lessons from animals with hyperinsulinaemia. Diabetes Metab 1996;22:122–131.

13 Zimmet P, Boyko EJ, Collier GR, de Courten M: Etiology of the metabolic syndrome: potential role of insulin resistance, leptin resistance, and other players. Ann NY Acad Sci 1999;892:25–44.

14 Hanley AJ, Wagenknecht LE, D'Agostino RB Jr, Zinman B, Haffner SM: Identification of subjects with insulin resistance and beta-cell dysfunction using alternative definitions of the metabolic syndrome. Diabetes 2003;52: 2740–2747.

15 Karter AJ, Mayer-Davis EJ, Selby JV, D'Agostino RB Jr, Haffner SM, Sholinsky P, Bergman R, Saad MF, Hamman RF: Insulin sensitivity and abdominal obesity in African-American, Hispanic, and non-Hispanic white men and women. The Insulin Resistance and Atherosclerosis Study. Diabetes 1996;45:1547–1555.

16 Howard BV, Mayer-Davis EJ, Goff D, Zaccaro DJ, Laws A, Robbins DC, Saad MF, Selby J, Hamman RF, Krauss RM, Haffner SM: Relationships between insulin resistance and lipoproteins in nondiabetic African Americans, Hispanics, and non-Hispanic whites: the Insulin Resistance Atherosclerosis Study. Metabolism 1998;47:1174–1179.

17 Ford ES, Giles WH, Dietz WH: Prevalence of the metabolic syndrome among US adults: findings from the third National Health and Nutrition Examination Survey. JAMA 2002; 287:356–359.

18 Athyros VG, Ganotakis ES, Elisaf M, Mikhailidis DP: The prevalence of the metabolic syndrome using the National Cholesterol Educational Program and International Diabetes Federation definitions. Curr Med Res Opin 2005;21:1157–1159.

19 Lawlor DA, Smith GD, Ebrahim S: Does the new International Diabetes Federation definition of the metabolic syndrome predict CHD any more strongly than older definitions? Findings from the British Women's Heart and Health Study. Diabetologia 2006; 49:41–48.

20 Eckel RH, Grundy SM, Zimmet PZ: The metabolic syndrome. Lancet 2005;365:1415–1428.

21 Sandhofer A, Iglseder B, Paulweber B, Ebenbichler CF, Patsch JR: Comparison of different definitions of the metabolic syndrome. Eur J Clin Invest 2007;37:109–116.

22 Ford ES, Giles WH, Mokdad AH: Increasing prevalence of the metabolic syndrome among US adults. Diabetes 2004;27:2444–2449.

23 Joost HG, Gibney MJ, Cashman KD, Gorman U, Hesketh JE, Mueller M, van Ommen B, Williams CM, Mathers JC: Personalised nutrition: status and perspectives. Br J Nutr 2007;98:26–31.

24 Freeman MS, Mansfield MJ, Barrett JH, Grant PJ: Heritability of features of the insulin resistance syndrome in a community-based study of healthy families. Diabet Med 2002;19:994–999.

25 Mills GW, Avery PJ, McCarthy MI, Hattersley AT, Levy JC, Hitman GA, Sampson M, Walker M: Heritability estimates for beta cell function and features of the insulin resistance syndrome in UK families with an increased susceptibility to type 2 diabetes. Diabetologia 2004;47:732–738.

26 Poulsen P, Vaag A, Kyvik K, Beck-Nielsen H: Genetic versus environmental aetiology of the metabolic syndrome among male and female twins. Diabetologia 2001;44:537–543.

27 Poulsen P, Levin K, Petersen I, Christensen K, Beck-Nielsen H, Vaag A: Heritability of insulin secretion, peripheral and hepatic insulin action, and intracellular glucose partitioning in young and old Danish twins. Diabetes 2005;54:275–283.

28 Grant SF, Thorleifsson G, Reynisdottir I, Benediktsson R, Manolescu A, Sainz J, Helgason A, Stefansson H, Emilsson V, Helgadottir A, Styrkarsdottir U, Magnusson KP, Walters GB, Palsdottir E, Jonsdottir T, Gudmundsdottir T, Gylfason A, Saemundsdottir J, Wilensky RL, Reilly MP, Rader DJ, Bagger Y, Christiansen C, Gudnason V, Sigurdsson G, Thorsteinsdottir U, Gulcher JR, Kong A, Stefansson K: Variant of transcription factor 7-like 2 (TCF7L2) gene confers risk of type 2 diabetes. Nat Genet 2006;38:320–323.

29 Florez JC, Jablonski KA, Bayley N, Pollin TI, de Bakker PI, Shuldiner AR, Knowler WC, Nathan DM, Altshuler D; Diabetes Prevention Program Research Group: TCF7L2 polymorphisms and progression to diabetes in the Diabetes Prevention Program. N Engl J Med 2006;355:241–250.

30 Wang J, Kuusisto J, Vänttinen M, Kuulasmaa T, Lindström J, Tuomilehto J, Uusitupa M, Laakso M: Variants of transcription factor 7-like 2 (TCF7L2) gene predict conversion to type 2 diabetes in the Finnish Diabetes Prevention Study and are associated with impaired glucose regulation and impaired insulin secretion. Diabetologia 2007;50: 1192–1200.

31 Sladek R, Rocheleau G, Rung J, Dina C, Shen L, Serre D, Boutin P, Vincent D, Belisle A, Hadjadj S, Balkau B, Heude B, Charpentier G, Hudson TJ, Montpetit A, Pshezhetsky AV, Prentki M, Posner BI, Balding DJ, Meyre D, Polychronakos C, Froguel P: A genome-wide association study identifies novel risk loci for type 2 diabetes. Nature 2007;445:881–885.

32 Steinthorsdottir V, Thorleifsson G, Reynisdottir I, Benediktsson R, Jonsdottir T, Walters GB, Styrkarsdottir U, Gretarsdottir S, Emilsson V, Ghosh S, Baker A, Snorradottir S, Bjarnason H, Ng MC, Hansen T, Bagger Y, Wilensky RL, Reilly MP, Adeyemo A, Chen Y, Zhou J, Gudnason V, Chen G, Huang H, Lashley K, Doumatey A, So WY, Ma RC, Andersen G, Borch-Johnsen K, Jorgensen T, van Vliet-Ostaptchouk JV, Hofker MH, Wijmenga C, Christiansen C, Rader DJ, Rotimi C, Gurney M, Chan JC, Pedersen O, Sigurdsson G, Gulcher JR, Thorsteinsdottir U, Kong A, Stefansson K: A variant in CDKAL1 influences insulin response and risk of type 2 diabetes. Nat Genet 2007;39:770–775.

33 Wei FY, Nagashima K, Ohshima T, Saheki Y, Lu YF, Matsushita M, Yamada Y, Mikoshiba K, Seino Y, Matsui H, Tomizawa K: Cdk5-dependent regulation of glucose-stimulated insulin secretion. Nat Med 2005;11:1104–1108.
34 Frayling TM, Timpson NJ, Weedon MN, Zeggini E, Freathy RM, Lindgren CM, Perry JR, Elliott KS, Lango H, Rayner NW, Shields B, Harries LW, Barrett JC, Ellard S, Groves CJ, Knight B, Patch AM, Ness AR, Ebrahim S, Lawlor DA, Ring SM, Ben-Shlomo Y, Jarvelin MR, Sovio U, Bennett AJ, Melzer D, Ferrucci L, Loos RJ, Barroso I, Wareham NJ, Karpe F, Owen KR, Cardon LR, Walker M, Hitman GA, Palmer CN, Doney AS, Morris AD, Smith GD, Hattersley AT, McCarthy MI: A common variant in the FTO gene is associated with body mass index and predisposes to childhood and adult obesity. Science 2007;316:889–894.
35 Silander K, Mohlke KL, Scott LJ, Peck EC, Hollstein P, Skol AD, Jackson AU, Deloukas P, Hunt S, Stavrides G, Chines PS, Erdos MR, Narisu N, Conneely KN, Li C, Fingerlin TE, Dhanjal SK, Valle TT, Bergman RN, Tuomilehto J, Watanabe RM, Boehnke M, Collins FS: Genetic variation near the hepatocyte nuclear factor-4 alpha gene predicts susceptibility to type 2 diabetes. Diabetes 2004;53:1141–1149.
36 Pajukanta P, Nuotio I, Terwilliger JD, Porkka KV, Ylitalo K, Pihlajamaki J, Suomalainen AJ, Syvanen AC, Lehtimaki T, Viikari JS, Laakso M, Taskinen MR, Ehnholm C, Peltonen L: Linkage of familial combined hyperlipidaemia to chromosome 1q21-q23. Nat Genet 1998;18:369–373.
37 Das SK, Hasstedt SJ, Zhang Z, Elbein SC: Linkage and association mapping of a chromosome 1q21-q24 type 2 diabetes susceptibility locus in northern European Caucasians. Diabetes 2004;53:492–499.
38 Xiang K, Wang Y, Zheng T, Jia W, Li J, Chen L, Shen K, Wu S, Lin X, Zhang G, Wang C, Wang S, Lu H, Fang Q, Shi Y, Zhang R, Xu J, Weng Q: Genome-wide search for type 2 diabetes/impaired glucose homeostasis susceptibility genes in the Chinese: significant linkage to chromosome 6q21-q23 and chromosome 1q21-q24. Diabetes 2004;53:228–234.
39 Horikawa Y, Oda N, Cox NJ, Li X, Orho-Melander M, Hara M, Hinokio Y, Lindner TH, Mashima H, Schwarz PE, del Bosque-Plata L, Horikawa Y, Oda Y, Yoshiuchi I, Colilla S, Polonsky KS, Wei S, Concannon P, Iwasaki N, Schulze J, Baier LJ, Bogardus C, Groop L, Boerwinkle E, Hanis CL, Bell GI: Genetic variation in the gene encoding calpain-10 is associated with type 2 diabetes mellitus. Nat Genet 2000;26:163–175.
40 Florez JC, Hirschhorn J, Altshuler D: The inherited basis of diabetes mellitus: implications for the genetic analysis of complex traits. Annu Rev Genomics Hum Genet 2003;4:257–291.
41 Gloyn AL: The search for type 2 diabetes genes. Ageing Res Rev 2003;2:111–127.
42 Bento JL, Palmer ND, Mychaleckyj JC, Lange LA, Langefeld CD, Rich SS, Freedman BI, Bowden DW: Association of protein tyrosine phosphatase 1B gene polymorphisms with type 2 diabetes. Diabetes 2004;53:3007–3012.
43 Palmer ND, Bento JL, Mychaleckyj JC, Langefeld CD, Campbell JK, Norris JM, Haffner SM, Bergman RN, Bowden DW; Insulin Resistance Atherosclerosis Study (IRAS) Family Study: Association of protein tyrosine phosphatase 1B gene polymorphisms with measures of glucose homeostasis in Hispanic Americans: the insulin resistance atherosclerosis study (IRAS) family study. Diabetes 2004;53:3013–3019.
44 Barthel A, Schmoll D: Novel concepts in insulin regulation of hepatic gluconeogenesis. Am J Physiol Endocrinol Metab 2003;285: E685–E692.
45 George S, Rochford JJ, Wolfrum C, Gray SL, Schinner S, Wilson JC, Soos MA, Murgatroyd PR, Williams RM, Acerini CL, Dunger DB, Barford D, Umpleby AM, Wareham NJ, Davies HA, Schafer AJ, Stoffel M, O'Rahilly S, Barroso I: A family with severe insulin resistance and diabetes due to a mutation in AKT2. Science 2004;304:1325–1328.
46 Puigserver P, Rhee J, Donovan J, Walkey CJ, Yoon JC, Oriente F, Kitamura Y, Altomonte J, Dong H, Accili D, Spiegelman BM: Insulin-regulated hepatic gluconeogenesis through FOXO1-PG 1alpha interaction. Nature 2003;423:550–555.
47 Sesti S: Pathophysiology of insulin resistance. Best Pract Res Clin Endocrinol Metab 2006;20:665–679.
48 Barak Y, Nelson MC, Ong ES, Jones YZ, Ruiz-Lozano P, Chien KR, Koder A, Evans RM: PPAR gamma is required for placental, cardiac, and adipose tissue development. Mol Cell 1999;4:585–595.
49 Barroso I, Gurnell M, Crowley VE, Agostini M, Schwabe JW, Soos MA, Maslen GL, Williams TD, Lewis H, Schafer AJ, Chatterjee VK, O'Rahilly S: Dominant negative mutations in human PPARgamma associated with severe insulin resistance, diabetes mellitus and hypertension. Nature 1999;402: 880–883.
50 Gurnell M: PPARgamma and metabolism: insights from the study of human genetic variants. Clin Endocrinol 2003;59:267–277.
51 Deeb SS, Fajas L, Nemoto M, Pihlajamaki J, Mykkanen L, Kuusisto J, Laakso M, Fujimoto W, Auwerx J: A Pro12Ala substitution in PPARgamma2 associated with decreased receptor activity, lower body mass index and improved insulin sensitivity. Nat Genet 1998;20:284–287.
52 Mancini FP, Vaccaro O, Sabatino L, Tufano A, Rivellese AA, Riccardi G, Colantuoni V: Pro12Ala substitution in the peroxisome proliferator-activated receptor-g2 is not associated with type 2 diabetes. Diabetes 1999; 48:1466–1468.
53 Clement K, Hercberg S, Passinge B, Galan P, Varroud-Vial M, Shuldiner AR, Beamer BA, Charpentier G, Guy-Grand B, Froguel P, Vaisse C: The Pro115Gln and Pro12Ala PPARg gene mutations in obesity and type 2 diabetes. Int J Obes Relat Metab Disord 2000; 24:391–393.
54 Ringel J, Engeli S, Distler A, Sharma AM: Pro12Ala missense mutation of the peroxisome proliferator activated receptor gamma and diabetes mellitus. Biochem Biophys Res Commun 1999;254:450–453.
55 Meirhaeghe A, Fajas L, Helbecque N, Cottel D, Auwerx J, Deeb SS, Amouyel P: Impact of the peroxisome proliferator activated receptor g2 Pro12Ala polymorphism on adiposity, lipids and non-insulin-dependent diabetes mellitus. Int J Obes Relat Metab Disord 2000; 24:195–199.
56 Hara K, Okada T, Tobe K, Yasuda K, Mori Y, Kadowaki H, Hagura R, Akanuma Y, Kimura S, Ito C, Kadowaki T: The Pro12Ala polymorphism in PPARg2 may confer resistance to type 2 diabetes. Biochem Biophys Res Commun 2000;271:212–216.
57 Altshuler D, Hirschhorn JN, Klannemark M, Lindgren CM, Vohl MC, Nemesh J, Lindgren CM, Vohl MC, Nemesh J, Lane CR, Schaffner SF, Bolk S, Brewer C, Tuomi T, Gaudet D, Hudson TJ, Daly M, Groop L, Lander ES: The common PPARgamma Pro12Ala polymorphism is associated with decreased risk of type 2 diabetes. Nat Genet 2000;26:76–80.
58 Ghoussaini M, Meyre D, Lobbens S, Charpentier G, Clement K, Charles MA, Tauber M, Weill J, Froguel P : Implication of the Pro-12Ala polymorphism of the PPAR-gamma 2 gene in type 2 diabetes and obesity in the French population. BMC Med Genet 2005;6: 11.
59 Andrulionyte L, Zacharova J, Chiasson JL, Laakso M; STOP-NIDDM Study Group: Common polymorphisms of the PPAR-gamma2 (Pro12Ala) and PGC-1alpha (Gly482Ser) genes are associated with the conversion from impaired glucose tolerance to type 2 diabetes in the STOP-NIDDM trial. Diabetologia 2004;47:2176–2184.
60 Doney AS, Fischer B, Cecil JE, Boylan K, McGuigan FE, Ralston SH, Morris AD, Palmer CN: Association of the Pro12Ala and C1431T variants of PPARG and their haplotypes with susceptibility to Type 2 diabetes. Diabetologia 2004;47:555–558.
61 Meirhaeghe A, Cottel D, Amouyel P, Dallongeville J: Association between peroxisome proliferator-activated receptor gamma haplotypes and the metabolic syndrome in French men and women. Diabetes 2005;54: 3043–3048.

62 Acton S, Osgood D, Donoghue M, Corella D, Pocovi M, Cenarro A, Mozas P, Keilty J, Squazzo S, Woolf EA, Ordovas JM: Association of polymorphisms at the SR-BI gene locus with plasma lipid levels and body mass index in a white population. Arterioscler Thromb Vasc Biol 1999;19:1734–1743.
63 Corella D, Guillen M, Saiz C, Portoles O, Sabater A, Folch J, Ordovas JM: Associations of LPL and APOC3 gene polymorphisms on plasma lipids in a Mediterranean population: interaction with tobacco smoking and the APOE locus. J Lipid Res 2002;43:416–427.
64 Hutter CM, Austin MA, Farin FM, Viernes HM, Edwards KL, Leonetti DL, McNeely MJ, Fujimoto WY: Association of endothelial lipase gene (LIPG) haplotypes with high-density lipoprotein cholesterol subfractions and apolipoprotein AI plasma levels in Japanese Americans. Atherosclerosis 2006;185:78–86.
65 Deeb SS, Zambon A, Carr MC, Ayyobi AF, Brunzell JD: Hepatic lipase and dyslipidemia: interactions among genetic variants, obesity, gender, and diet. J Lipid Res 2003;44:1279–1286.
66 Talmud PJ, Hawe E, Martin S, Olivier M, Miller GJ, Rubin EM, Pennacchio LA, Humphries SE: Relative contribution of variation within the APOC3/A4/A5 gene cluster in determining plasma triglycerides. Hum Mol Genet 2002;11:3039–3046.
67 Lai CQ, Demissie S, Cupples LA, Zhu Y, Adiconis X, Parnell LD, Corella D, Ordovas JM: Influence of the APOA5 locus on plasma triglyceride, lipoprotein subclasses, and CVD risk in the Framingham Heart Study. J Lipid Res 2004;45:2096–2105.
68 Mar R, Pajukanta P, Allayee H, Groenendijk M, Dallinga-Thie G, Krauss RM, Sinsheimer JS, Cantor RM, de Bruin TW, Lusis AJ: Association of the APOLIPOPROTEIN A1/C3/A4/A5 gene cluster with triglyceride levels and LDL particle size in familial combined hyperlipidemia. Circ Res 2004;94:993–999.
69 Guettier JM, Georgopoulos A, Tsai MY, Radha V, Shanthirani S, Deepa R, Gross M, Rao G, Mohan V: Polymorphisms in the fatty acid-binding protein 2 and apolipoprotein C-III genes are associated with the metabolic syndrome and dyslipidemia in a South Indian population. J Clin Endocrinol Metab 2005;90:1705–1711.
70 Hirschhorn JN, Lohmueller K, Byrne E, Hirschhorn K: A comprehensive review of genetic association studies. Genet Med 2002;4:45–61.
71 Boden, G: Role of fatty acids in the pathogenesis of insulin resistance and NIDDM. Diabetes 1997;46:3–10.
72 Reaven GM, Hollenbeck C, Jeng CY, Wu MS, Chen YD: Measurement of plasma glucose, free fatty acid, lactate, and insulin for 24 h in patients with NIDDM. Diabetes 1988;37:1020–1024.
73 Randle PJ, Garland PB, Hales CN, Newsholme EA: The glucose fatty-acid cycle. Its role in insulin sensitivity and the metabolic disturbances of diabetes mellitus. Lancet 1963;1:785–789.
74 McGarry JD: Banting Lecture 2001: dysregulation of fatty acid metabolism in the etiology of type 2 diabetes. Diabetes 2002;51:7–18.
75 Prentki M, Corkey BE: Are the beta-cell signaling molecules malonyl-CoA and cystolic long-chain acyl-CoA implicated in multiple tissue defects of obesity and NIDDM? Diabetes 1996;45:273–283.
76 McGarry JD, Mannaerts GP, Foster DW: A possible role for malonyl-CoA in the regulation of hepatic fatty acid oxidation and ketogenesis. J Clin Invest 1977;60:265–270.
77 Stein DT, Esser V, Stevenson BE, Lane KE, Whiteside JH, Daniels MB, Chen S, McGarry JD: Essentiality of circulating fatty acids for glucose-stimulated insulin secretion in the fasted rat. J Clin Invest 1996;97:2728–2775.
78 Shimabukuro M, Zhou YT, Levi M, Unger RH: Fatty acid-induced beta cell apoptosis: a link between obesity and diabetes. Proc Natl Acad Sci USA 1998;95:2498–2502.
79 Hotamisligil GS, Peraldi P, Budavari A, Ellis R, White MF, Spiegelman BM: IRS-1-mediated inhibition of insulin receptor tyrosine kinase activity in TNF-alpha- and obesity-induced insulin resistance. Science 1996;271:665–668.
80 Shulman GI: Cellular mechanisms of insulin resistance. J Clin Invest 2000;106:171–176.
81 Gletsu NA, Clandinin MT: Impact of dietary fatty acid composition on insulin action at the nucleus. Ann NY Acad Sci 1997;827:188–199.
82 Field CJ, Toyomizu M, Clandinin MT: Relationship between dietary fat, adipocyte membrane composition and insulin binding in the rat. J Nutr 1989;119:1483–1489.
83 Fickova M, Hubert P, Klimes I, Staedel C, Cremel G, Bohov P, Macho L: Dietary fish oil and olive oil improve the liver insulin receptor tyrosine kinase activity in high sucrose fed rats. Endocr Regul 1994;28:187–197.
84 Taouis M, Dagou C, Ster C, Durand G, Pinault M, Delarue J: N-3 polyunsaturated fatty acids prevent the defect of insulin receptor signaling in muscle. Am J Physiol Endocrinol Metab 2002;282:664–671.
85 Luo J, Rizkalla SW, Boillot J, Alamowitch C, Chaib H, Bruzzo F, Desplanque N, Dalix AM, Durand G, Slama G: Dietary (n-3) polyunsaturated fatty acids improve adipocyte insulin action and glucose metabolism in insulin-resistant rats: relation to membrane fatty acids. J Nutr 1996;126:1951–1958.
86 Hunnicutt JW, Hardy RW, Williford J, McDonald JM: Saturated fatty acid-induced insulin resistance in rat adipocytes. Diabetes 1994;43:540–545.
87 Hu FB, van Dam RM, Liu S: Diet and risk of type II diabetes: the role of types of fat and carbohydrate. Diabetologia 2001;44:805–817.
88 Vessby B, Unsitupa M, Hermansen K, Riccardi G, Rivellese AA, Tapsell LC, Nalsen C, Berglund L, Louheranta A, Rasmussen BM, Calvert GD, Maffetone A, Pedersen E, Gustafsson IB, Storlien LH: Substituting dietary saturated for monounsaturated fat impairs insulin sensitivity in healthy men and women: The KANWU Study. Diabetologia 2001;44:312–319.
89 Salas J, Lopez Miranda J, Jansen S, Zambrana JL, Castro P, Paniagua JA, Blanco A, Lopez Segura F, Jimenez Pereperez JA, Perez Jimenez F: The diet rich in monounsaturated fat modifies in a beneficial way carbohydrate metabolism and arterial pressure (in Spanish). Med Clin (Barc) 1999;113:765–769.
90 Parillo M, Rivellese AA, Ciardullo AV, Capaldo B, Giacco A, Genovese S, Riccardi G: A high-monounsaturated-fat/low-carbohydrate diet improves peripheral insulin sensitivity in non-insulin-dependent diabetic patients. Metabolism 1992;41:1373–1378.
91 Lovejoy JC, Smith SR, Champagne CM, Most MM, Lefevre M, DeLany JP, Denkins YM, Rood JC, Veldhuis J, Bray GA: Effects of diets enriched in saturated (palmitic), monounsaturated (oleic), or trans (elaidic) fatty acids on insulin sensitivity and substrate oxidation in healthy adults. Diabetes Care 2002;25:1283–1288.
92 Berry EM: Who's afraid of n-6 polyunsaturated fatty acids? Methodological considerations for assessing whether they are harmful. Nutr Metab Cardiovasc Dis 2001;11:181–188.
93 van Dam RM, Willett WC, Rimm EB, Stampfer MJ, Hu FB: Dietary fat and meat intake in relation to risk of type 2 diabetes in men. Diabetes Care 2002;25:417–424.
94 West KM, Kalbfleisch JM: Influence of nutritional factors on prevalence of diabetes. Diabetes 1971;20:99–108.
95 Wang L, Folsom AR, Zheng ZJ, Pankow JS, Eckfeldt JH: Plasma fatty acid composition and incidence of diabetes in middle-aged adults: the Atherosclerosis Risk in Communities (ARIC) Study. Am J Clin Nutr 2003;78:91–98.
96 Meyer KA, Kushi LH, Jacobs DR Jr, Folsom AR: Dietary fat and incidence of type 2 diabetes in older Iowa women. Diabetes Care 2001;24:1528–35.
97 Ryan M, McInerney D, Owens D, Collins P, Johnson A, Tomkin GH: Diabetes and the Mediterranean diet: a beneficial effect of oleic acid on insulin sensitivity, adipocyte glucose transport and endothelium-dependent vasoreactivity. QJM 2000;93:85–91.
98 Soriguer F, Esteva I, Rojo-Martinez G, Ruiz de Adana MS, Dobarganes M C, Garcia-Almeida JM, Tinahones F, Beltran M, Gonzalez-Romero S, Olveira G, Gomez-Zumaquero JM: Oleic acid from cooking oils is associated with lower insulin resistance in the general population (Pizarra study). Eur J Endocrinol 2004;150:33–39.

99 Mayer-Davis EJ, Monaco JH, Hoen HM, Carmichael S, Vitolins MZ, Rewers MJ, Haffner SM, Ayad MF, Bergman RN, Karter AJ: Dietary fat and insulin sensitivity in a triethnic population: the role of obesity. The Insulin Resistance Atherosclerosis Study (IRAS). Am J Clin Nutr 1997;65:79–87.
100 Consensus Development Conference on Diet and Exercise in Non-Insulin-Dependent Diabetes Mellitus. National Institutes of Health. Diabetes Care 1987;10:639–644.
101 Heine RJ, Mulder C, Popp-Snijders C, van der Meer J, van der Veen EA: Linoleic-acid-enriched diet: long-term effects on serum lipoprotein and apolipoprotein concentrations and insulin sensitivity in noninsulin-dependent diabetic patients. Am J Clin Nutr 1989;49:448–456.
102 Storlien LH, Baur LA, Kriketos AD, Pan DA, Cooney GJ, Jenkins AB, Calvert GD, Campbell LV: Dietary fats and insulin action. Diabetologia 1996;39:621–631.
103 Storlien LH, Jenkins AB, Chisholm DJ, Pascoe WS, Khouri S, Kraegen EW: Influence of dietary fat composition on development of insulin resistance in rats. Relationship to muscle triglyceride and omega-3 fatty acids in muscle phospholipids. Diabetes 1991; 40:280–289.
104 Laaksonen DE, Lakka TA, Lakka HM, Nyyssonen K, Rissanen T, Niskanen LK, Salonen JT: Serum fatty acid composition predicts development of impaired fasting glycaemia and diabetes in middle-aged men. Diabet Med 2002;19:456–464.
105 Salmeron J, Hu FB, Manson JE, Stampfer MJ, Colditz GA, Rimm EB, Willett WC: Dietary fat intake and risk of type 2 diabetes in women. Am J Clin Nutr 2001;73:1019–1026.
106 Somova L, Moodley K, Channa ML, Nadar A: Dose-dependent effect of dietary fish-oil (n-3) polyunsaturated fatty acids on in vivo insulin sensitivity in rat. Methods Find Exp Clin Pharmacol 1999;21:275–278.
107 Pan DA, Lillioja S, Milner MR, Kriketos AD, Baur LA, Bogardus C, Storlien LH: Skeletal muscle membrane lipid composition is related to adiposity and insulin action. J Clin Invest 1995;96:2802–2808.
108 Borkman M, Storlien LH, Pan DA, Jenkins AB, Chisholm DJ, Campbell LV: The relation between insulin sensitivity and the fatty-acid composition of skeletal-muscle phospholipids. N Engl J Med 1993;328:238–244.
109 Connor SL, Connor WE: Are fish oils beneficial in the prevention and treatment of coronary artery disease? Am J Clin Nutr 1997;66:1020S–1031S.
110 Feskens EJ, Virtanen SM, Rasanen L, Tuomilehto J, Stengard J, Pekkanen J, Nissinen A, Kromhout D: Dietary factors determining diabetes and impaired glucose tolerance. A 20-year follow-up of the Finnish and Dutch cohorts of the Seven Countries Study. Diabetes Care 1995;18:1104–1112.
111 Feskens EJ, Loeber JG, Kromhout D: Diet and physical activity as determinants of hyperinsulinemia: the Zutphen Elderly Study. Am J Epidemiol 1994;140:350–360.
112 Fukagawa NK, Anderson JW, Hageman G, Young VR, Minaker KL: High-carbohydrate, high-fiber diets increase peripheral insulin sensitivity in healthy young and old adults. Am J Clin Nutr 1990;52:524–528.
113 Chen M, Bergman RN, Porte D Jr: Insulin resistance and beta-cell dysfunction in aging: the importance of dietary carbohydrate. J Clin Endocrinol Metab 1988;67: 951–957.
114 Lovejoy JC, Windhauser MM, Rood JC, de la Bretonne JA: Effect of a controlled high-fat versus low-fat diet on insulin sensitivity and leptin levels in African-American and Caucasian women. Metabolism 1998;47: 1520–1524.
115 Vessby B: Dietary fat and insulin action in humans. Br J Nutr 2000;83(suppl 1):S91–S6.
116 Vessby B, Tengblad S, Lithell H: Insulin sensitivity is related to the fatty acid composition of serum lipids and skeletal muscle phospholipids in 70-year-old men. Diabetologia 1994;37:1044–1050.
117 Warensjo E, Ohrvall M, Vessby B: Fatty acid composition and estimated desaturase activities are associated with obesity and lifestyle variables in men and women. Nutr Metab Cardiovasc Dis 2006;16:128–136.
118 Warensjo E, Sundstrom J, Lind L, Vessby B: Factor analysis of fatty acids in serum lipids as a measure of dietary fat quality in relation to the metabolic syndrome in men. Am J Clin Nutr 2006;84:442–448.
119 Ordovas JM, Corella D: Nutritional genomics. Annu Rev Genomics Hum Genet 2004; 5:71–118.
120 Perez-Jimenez E, Lopez-Miranda J, Pinillos MD, Gomez P, Paz-Rojas E, Montilla P, Marin C, Velasco MJ, Blanco-Molina A, Jimenez Pereperez JA, Ordovas JM: A Mediterranean and a high-carbohydrate diet improve glucose metabolism in healthy young persons. Diabetologia 2001;44:2038–2043.
121 Bos G, Snijder MB, Nijpels G, Dekker JM, Stehouwer CD, Bouter LM, Heine RJ, Jansen H: Opposite contributions of trunk and leg fat mass with plasma lipase activities: the Hoorn study. Obes Res 2005;13:1817–1823.
122 Santos JL, Boutin P, Verdich C, Holst C, Larsen LH, Toubro S, Dina C, Saris WH, Blaak EE, Hoffstedt J, Taylor MA, Polak J, Clement K, Langin D, Astrup A, Froguel P, Pedersen O, Sorensen TI, Martinez JA; The NUGENOB Consortium: Genotype-by-nutrient interactions assessed in European obese women: a case-only study. Eur J Nutr 2006;45:454–462.
123 Ordovas JM, Corella D, Demissie S, Cupples LA, Couture P, Coltell O, Wilson PW, Schaefer EJ, Tucker KL: Dietary fat intake determines the effect of a common polymorphism in the hepatic lipase gene promoter on high-density lipoprotein metabolism: evidence of a strong dose effect in this gene-nutrient interaction in the Framingham Study. Circulation 2002;106:2315–2231.
124 Elosua R, Ordovas JM, Cupples LA, Lai CQ, Demissie S, Fox CS, Polak JF, Wolf PA, D'Agostino RB Sr, O'Donnell CJ: Variants at the APOA5 locus, association with carotid atherosclerosis, and modification by obesity: the Framingham Study. J Lipid Res 2006;47:990–996.
125 Lai CQ, Corella D, Demissie S, Cupples LA, Adiconis X, Zhu Y, Parnell LD, Tucker KL, Ordovas JM: Dietary intake of n-6 fatty acids modulates effect of apolipoprotein A5 gene on plasma fasting triglycerides, remnant lipoprotein concentrations, and lipoprotein particle size: the Framingham Heart Study. Circulation 2006;113:2062–2070.
126 Corella D, Lai CQ, Demissie S, Cupples LA, Manning AK, Tucker KL, Ordovas JM: APOA5 gene variation modulates the effects of dietary fat intake on body mass index and obesity risk in the Framingham Heart Study J Mol Med 2007;85:119–128.
127 Olivieri O, Martinelli N, Sandri M, Bassi A, Guarini P, Trabetti E, Pizzolo F, Girelli D, Friso S, Pignatti PF, Corrocher R: Apolipoprotein C-III, n-3 polyunsaturated fatty acids, and 'insulin-resistant' T-455C APOC3 gene polymorphism in heart disease patients: example of gene-diet interaction. Clin Chem 2005;51:360–367.
128 Moreno JA, Lopez-Miranda J, Marin C, Gomez P, Perez-Martinez P, Fuentes F, Fernandez de la Puebla RA, Paniagua JA, Ordovas JM, Perez-Jimenez F: The influence of the apolipoprotein E gene promoter (–219G/T) polymorphism on postprandial lipoprotein metabolism in young normolipemic males. J Lipid Res 2003;44:2059–2064.
129 Moreno JA, Perez-Jimenez F, Marin C, Gomez P, Perez-Martinez P, Moreno R, Bellido C, Fuentes F, Lopez-Miranda J: Apolipoprotein E gene promoter –219G→T polymorphism increases LDL-cholesterol concentrations and susceptibility to oxidation in response to a diet rich in saturated fat. Am J Clin Nutr 2004;80:1404–1409.
130 Moreno JA, Perez-Jimenez F, Marin C, Perez-Martinez P, Moreno R, Gomez P, Jimenez-Gomez Y, Paniagua JA, Lairon D, Lopez-Miranda J: The apolipoprotein E gene promoter (–219G/T) polymorphism determines insulin sensitivity in response to dietary fat in healthy young adults. J Nutr 2005;135:2535–2540.

131 Perez-Martinez P, Lopez-Miranda J, Ordovas JM, Bellido C, Marin C, Gomez P, Paniagua JA, Moreno JA, Fuentes F, Perez-Jimenez F: Postprandial lipemia is modified by the presence of the polymorphism present in the exon 1 variant at the SR-BI gene locus. J Mol Endocrinol 2004;32:237–245.

132 Perez-Martinez P, Perez-Jimenez F, Bellido C, Ordovas JM, Moreno JA, Marin C, Gomez P, Delgado-Lista J, Fuentes F, Lopez-Miranda J: A polymorphism exon 1 variant at the locus of the scavenger receptor class B type I (SCARB1) gene is associated with differences in insulin sensitivity in healthy people during the consumption of an olive oil-rich diet. J Clin Endocrinol Metab 2005;90:2297–2300.

133 Marin C, Perez-Jimenez F, Gomez P, Delgado J, Paniagua JA, Lozano A, Cortes B, Jimenez-Gomez Y, Gomez MJ, Lopez-Miranda J: The Ala54Thr polymorphism of the fatty acid-binding protein 2 gene is associated with a change in insulin sensitivity after a change in the type of dietary fat. Am J Clin Nutr 2005;82:196–200.

134 Neschen S, Morino K, Dong J, Wang-Fischer Y, Cline GW, Romanelli AJ, Rossbacher JC, Moore IK, Regittnig W, Munoz DS, Kim JH, Shulman GI: n–3 Fatty acids preserve insulin sensitivity in vivo in a peroxisome proliferator-activated receptor-alpha-dependent manner. Diabetes 2007;56:1034–1041.

135 Tai ES, Corella D, Demissie S, Cupples LA, Coltell O, Schaefer EJ, Tucker KL, Ordovas JM; Framingham Heart Study: Polyunsaturated fatty acids interact with the PPARA-L162V polymorphism to affect plasma triglyceride and apolipoprotein CIII concentrations in the Framingham Heart Study. J Nutr 2005;135:397–403.

136 Paradis AM, Fontaine-Bisson B, Bosse Y, Robitaille J, Lemieux S, Jacques H, Lamarche B, Tchernof A, Couture P, Vohl MC: The peroxisome proliferator-activated receptor alpha Leu162Val polymorphism influences the metabolic response to a dietary intervention altering fatty acid proportions in healthy men. Am J Clin Nutr 2005;81:523–530.

137 Stefan N, Wahl HG, Fritsche A, Harring H, Stumvoll M: Effect of the pattern of elevated free fatty acids on insulin sensitivity and insulin secretion in healthy humans. Horm Metab Res 2001;33:432–438.

138 Vessby B, Gustafsson IB, Tengblad S, Boberg M, Andersson A: Desaturation and elongation of fatty acids and insulin action. Ann NY Acad Sci 2002;967:183–195.

139 Luan J, Browne PO, Harding AH, Halsall DJ, O'Rahilly S, Chatterjee VK, Wareham NJ: Evidence for gene-nutrient interaction at the PPARgamma locus. Diabetes 2001;50:686–689.

140 Robitaille J, Despres JP, Perusse L, Vohl MC: The PPAR-gamma P12A polymorphism modulates the relationship between dietary fat intake and components of the metabolic syndrome: results from the Quebec Family Study. Clin Genet 2003;63:109–116.

141 Pisabarro RE, Sanguinetti C, Stoll M, Prendez D. High incidence of type 2 diabetes in peroxisome proliferators-activated receptor $\gamma 2$ Pro12Ala carriers exposed to a high chronic intake of trans fatty acids and saturated fatty acids. Diabetes Care 2004;27:2251–2252.

142 Tai ES, Corella D, Deurenberg-Yap M, Adiconis X, Chew SK, Tan CE, Ordovas JM: Differential effects of the C1431T and Pro12Ala PPARgamma gene variants on plasma lipids and diabetes risk in an Asian population. J Lipid Res 2004;45:674–685.

143 Lindi VI, Uusitupa MI, Lindstrom, Louheranta A, Eriksson JG, Valle TT, Hamalainen H, Ilanne-Parikka P, Keinanen-Kiukaanniemi S, Laakso M, Tuomilehto J; Finnish Diabetes Prevention Study: Association of the Pro12Ala polymorphism in the PPARgamma2 gene with 3-year incidence of type 2 diabetes and body weight change in the Finnish Diabetes Prevention Study. Diabetes 2002;51:2581–2586.

144 Scacchi R, Pinto A, Rickards O, Pacella A, De Stefano GF, Cannella C, Corbo RM: An analysis of peroxisome proliferator-activated receptor gamma (PPAR-gamma2) Pro12Ala polymorphism distribution and prevalence of type 2 diabetes mellitus (T2DM) in world populations in relation to dietary habits. Nutr Metab Cardiovasc Dis 2007[Epub ahead of print].

145 Harding HA, Day NE, Khaw KT, Bingham S, Luben R, Welsh A, Wareham NJ: Dietary fat and the risk of clinical type 2 diabetes. The European Prospective Investigation of Cancer-Norfolk Study. Am J Epidemiol 2004;159:73–82.

146 Franks PW, Luan J, Browne PO, Harding AH, O'Rahilly S, Chatterjee VK, Wareham NJ: Does peroxisome proliferator-activated receptor gamma genotype (Pro12ala) modify the association of physical activity and dietary fat with fasting insulin level? Metabolism 2004;53:11–16.

Journal of
Nutrigenetics
and
Nutrigenomics

Author Index Vol. 1, No. 3, 2008

Subject Index Vol. 1, No. 3, 2008

KARGER

Fax +41 61 306 12 34
E-Mail karger@karger.ch
www.karger.com

Accessible online at:
www.karger.com/jnn

International Society of Nutrigenetics / Nutrigenomics

Journal of Nutrigenetics and Nutrigenomics

Society News

Board of Directors 2008

Aims and Scope

The purpose of the society is to increase understanding through research and education of professionals and the general public of the role of genetic variation and dietary response and the role of nutrients in gene expression.

Next meeting

2nd Annual Congress of the International Society of Nutrigenetics and Nutrigenomics
Geneva, October 6–8, 2008
isnn2008@symporg.ch

Membership

Membership enquiries should be directed to:
S. Karger AG
Medical and Scientific Publishers
Attn: Mr. Peter Roth
Allschwilerstrasse 10
CH–4009 Basel (Switzerland)
Telefon +41 61 306 11 11
Fax +41 61 306 12 34
E-mail p.roth@karger.ch

Society Website

www.isnn.info

KI08601

ISNN

International Society of Nutrigenetics / Nutrigenomics

Please return this application to:
S. Karger AG
Medical and Scientific Publishers
Attn: Mr. Peter Roth
Allschwilerstrasse 10
CH–4009 Basel (Switzerland)
Tel. +41 61 306 1111
Fax +41 61 306 1234
E-mail p.roth@karger.ch

Membership Application for 2008

ISNN Executive Committee
President: Artemis P. Simopoulos, M.D. (USA)
Vice President: Raffaele De Caterina, M.D., Ph.D. (Italy)
Secretary: Philippa J. Talmud, Ph.D. (UK)
Treasurer: Jose Ordovas, Ph.D. (USA)

Membership is granted upon application and payment of annual membership dues. Membership is individual and non-transferable. Applicants may apply for either Regular or Associate Membership, as described below.

Regular Members. Membership in the ISNN is open to researchers, educators and clinicians, who have a continuing scientific interest in Nutrition and/or Genetics/Molecular Biology/Pharmacology. Regular members pay full annual dues, may nominate and vote in Society elections, may hold elected and appointed offices, may serve on committees, receive discounted registration for Society Congresses, and receive a complimentary subscription to the **Journal of Nutrigenetics and Nutrigenomics:** *Official Journal of the ISNN*, edited by Louis Pérusse, Ph.D. (Canada).

Associate Members must be students, trainees or post-doctoral fellows and may continue in Associate status for up to three years. Applicants must attach a letter from their institution or supervisor certifying their status. Associate Members pay reduced annual membership dues, may vote in Society matters, receive discounted registration to Society Congresses, serve on Committees and enjoy members-only privileges. Associate Members receive an online-only subscription to the Society's official journal.

Mailing address *(Please type or print legibly)*

Last name: ____________________
First name: ____________________
Title: ____________________
Current Professional Position: ____________________
Year of birth: ____________________
Department: ____________________
Institution: ____________________
Street Address: ____________________
City: ____________________
State/Province: __________ Zip Code: __________
Country: ____________________
Tel. #: __________ Fax#: __________
E-mail: ____________________

(Check all boxes that apply)

Degree:	**Affiliation:**	**Research Area:**
☐ MD	☐ Academic	☐ Nutrition
☐ PhD	☐ Industry	☐ Molecular Biology
☐ DSc	☐ Regulatory	☐ Genetics
☐	☐	☐ Pharmacology
		☐ Epidemiology
Specialties:		☐

INVOICE

☐ Regular Member for **2008**
(includes full subscription to the
Journal of Nutrigenetics and Nutrigenomics) .... US$ 200.00*

☐ Regular Member for **2008**
(includes online-only subscription to the
Journal of Nutrigenetics and Nutrigenomics) .... US$ 150.00

☐ Associate Member for **2008**:
student, fellow, trainee, technician**
(includes online-only subscription to the
Journal of Nutrigenetics and Nutrigenomics) .... US$ 90.00

** Includes $ 115 for the printed journal and online access plus $ 48 for postage and handling
** Please attach a letter from your institution verifying your status for 2007

☐ Corporation...................................... US$ 400.00

VOLUNTARY CONTRIBUTIONS .... US$ ______

TOTAL AMOUNT PAID .... **US$**

Payment by credit card only.
Please charge the total amount paid above to my credit card (check one):
☐ Visa ☐ MasterCard ☐ EuroCard ☐ American Express ☐ Diners

Name on card: ____________________
Card number: ____________________
Expiration date: ____________________
Authorized signature: ____________________

Please return this form to the address or fax number listed above.
Please note that dues are for the calendar year and are not prorated.

An excellent source of methodological and applied genetic research

Human Heredity

International Journal of Human and Medical Genetics

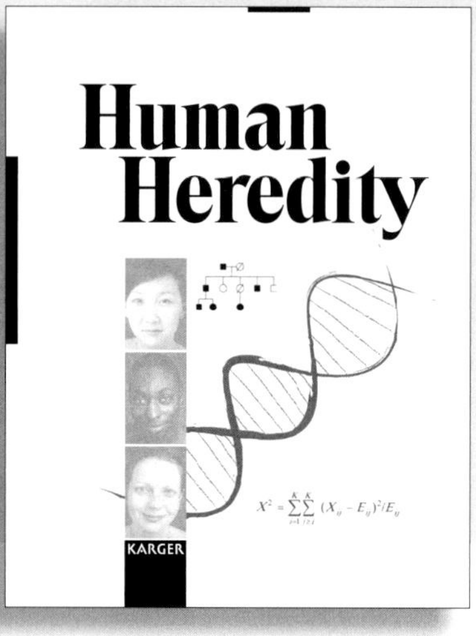

Gathering original research reports and short communications from all over the world, *Human Heredity* is devoted to methodological and applied research on the genetics of human populations, linkage analysis, genetic mechanisms of disease, and new methods in molecular and statistical genetics. The value of this information to many branches of medicine is shown by the number of citations the journal receives in fields ranging from immunology and hematology to epidemiology and public health planning, and the fact that at least 50% of all *Human Heredity* papers are still cited more than 8 years after publication (according to ISI Journal Citation Reports).

Selected contributions

Adaptive Two-Stage Analysis of Genetic Association in Case-Control Designs: **Zheng, G.** (Bethesda, Md.); **Song, K.** (King of Prussia, Pa.); **Elston, R.C.** (Cleveland, Ohio)

Evidence for a Locus in 1p31 Region Specifically Linked to the Co-Morbidity of Asthma and Allergic Rhinitis in the EGEA Study: **Dizier, M.-H.** (Villejuif); **Bouzigon, E.** (Evry); **Guilloud-Bataille, M.; Genin, E.; Oryszczyn, M.-P.** (Villejuif); **Annesi-Maesano, I.** (Paris); **Demenais, F.** (Evry)

Detection of Gene × Gene Interactions in Genome-Wide Association Studies of Human Population Data: **Musani, S.K.; Shriner, D.; Liu, N.; Feng, R.; Coffey, C.S.; Yi, N.; Tiwari, H.K.; Allison, D.B.** (Birmingham, Ala.)

Subsets of Finns with High HDL to Total Cholesterol Ratio Show Evidence for Linkage to Type 2 Diabetes on Chromosome 6q: **Shtir, C.; Nagakawa, I.S.** (Los Angeles, Calif.); **Duren, W.L.; Conneely, K.N.; Scott, L.J.** (Ann Arbor, Mich.); **Silander, K.** (Bethesda, Md.); **Valle, T.T.** (Helsinki); **Tuomilehto, J.** (Helsinki/Seinäjoki); **Buchanan, T.A.; Bergman, R.N.** (Los Angeles, Calif.); **Collins, F.S.** (Bethesda, Md.); **Boehnke, M.** (Ann Arbor, Mich.); **Watanabe, R.M.** (Los Angeles, Calif.)

Linkage Disequilibrium and Haplotype Homozygosity in Population Samples Genotyped at a High Marker Density: **Wang, H.; Lin, C.-H.; Service, S.** (Los Angeles, Calif.); **Chen, Y.** (Champain, Ill.); **Freimer, N.; Sabatti, C.** (Los Angeles, Calif.) The international collaborative group on isolated populations

Data-Mining Methods as Useful Tools for Predicting Individual Drug Response: Application to *CYP2D6* Data: **Sabbagh, A.; Darlu, P.** (Villejuif)

Human Population Genetic Structure and Diversity Inferred from Polymorphic *L1 (LINE-1)* and *Alu* Insertions: **Witherspoon, D.J.; Marchani, E.E.; Watkins, W.S.; Ostler, C.T.; Wooding, S.P.** (Salt Lake City, Utah); **Anders, B.A.; Fowlkes, J.D.** (Baton Rouge, La.); **Boissinot, S.** (Flushing, N.Y.); **Furano, A.V.** (Bethesda, Md.); **Ray, D.A.** (Baton Rouge, La.); **Rogers, A.R.** (Salt Lake City, Utah); **Batzer, M.A.** (Baton Rouge, La.); **Jorde, L.B.** (Salt Lake City, Utah)

Quantification of the Power of Hardy-Weinberg Equilibrium Testing to Detect Genotyping Error: **Cox, D.G.; Kraft, P.** (Boston, Mass.)

More information at
www.karger.com/hhe

- Pay-per-View and Subscriber Access to Full Text
- Full Table of Contents
- Full Editorial Board
- Free Abstracts and Selected Articles
- Online Sample Issue
- Submission/Guidelines for Authors
- Subscription Details
- Free Alert Service
- Online Library Recommendation

Human Heredity
2008: Volumes 65, 66
4 issues per volume
Language: English
ISSN 0001–5652 (print)
ISSN 1423–0062 (online)

Listed in bibliographic services, including *Current Contents®/Life Sciences, MEDLINE, Biological Abstracts, EMBASE/Excerpta Medica.*

KF08038

KARGER